INHERITED HEMOGLOBIN DISORDERS

Edited by **Anjana Munshi**

Inherited Hemoglobin Disorders
http://dx.doi.org/10.5772/59742
Edited by Anjana Munshi

Contributors

Mehrdad Payandeh, Jorge Pena Siado, Julian Esteban Londono, Nadia Maria Sposi, Ahmed Mansour, Ahmad Darwish, Sohier Yahia, Rasha El-Ashry, Angi Adel, Sonja Pavlovic, Milena Ugrin, Maja Stojiljkovic, Jean Leandro Dos Santos, Thais Regina Ferreira Melo, Lucas Ercolin, Rafael Chelucci, Aylime Melchior, Carolina Lanaro, Man Chin Chung, Yan Su, Wenbin Qin, Qitu He, Ghada El-Kamah, Khalda Amr, Anjana Munshi

Published by InTech

Janeza Trdine 9, 51000 Rijeka, Croatia

Publishing Process Manager Iva Simcic

Technical Editor InTech DTP team

Cover InTech Design team

First published November, 2015

Printed in Croatia

Additional hard copies can be obtained from orders@intechopen.com

Inherited Hemoglobin Disorders, Edited by Anjana Munshi

p. cm.

ISBN 978-953-51-2198-5

For EU product safety concerns:
IN TECH d.o.o., Prolaz Marije Krucifikse Kozulić 3, 51000 Rijeka, Croatia,
info@intechopen.com or visit our website at intechopen.com.

Meet the editor

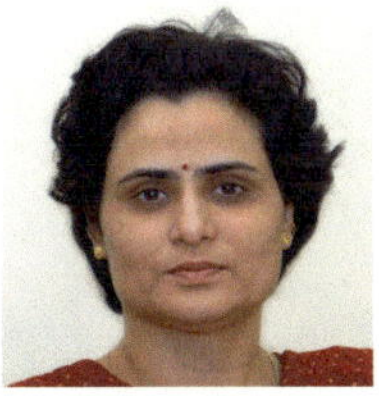

Anjana Munshi, M.Sc., M.Phil., Ph.D., is an Associate Professor, heading the Centre for Human Genetics and Molecular Medicine in the School of Health Sciences, Central University of Punjab, Bathinda, Punjab, India. Her expertise includes stroke genetics, hemoglobinopathies, pharmacogenetics, molecular cancer biology, epilepsy, and bioinformatics. Dr. Munshi has published 81 papers in international peer-reviewed journals and contributed 13 book chapters. She is a reviewer for several international research journals of global repute.

Contents

Preface

Hemoglobinopathies are the most prevalent genetically transmitted diseases worldwide, with an estimated 269 million carriers. Approximately 7% of the global population has been reported to be a carrier of hemoglobin disorders. Around 300,000–500,000 children are born annually with a severe hemoglobin disorder, out of which 80% are born in middle- and low-income countries. Most of the hemoglobinopathies are not clinically apparent, but some produce serious life-threatening diseases. The control of these syndromes poses a major challenge in clinical practice since these diseases occur in high prevalence, are lethal, and constitute a significant health-care burden. The thalassemias result from a wide variety of mutations in the alpha- and beta-globin genes that direct the synthesis of adult hemoglobin ($\alpha2\beta2$). Two major types of thalassemias, α and β respectively, are named after defects in these proteins coded by genes. Sickle cell disease (SCD) results from the substitution of glutamic acid by valine at the sixth position in the β-chain of hemoglobin. Every ethnic group or community has its own prevalence of the disease and spectrum of mutations causing these diseases. Current approaches of disease management include prenatal diagnosis, transfusion therapy, and bone marrow transplantation (BMT). BMT is potentially curative and has offered a definitive cure for a few patients.

The clinical expression of the disease is remarkably variable, ranging from nearly asymptomatic to severe, transfusion-dependent disease. However, what is not well understood is the marked variability of the clinical manifestations. The clinical picture in some patients may be a devastating course of acute and chronic events, resulting in severe end-organ damage, including pulmonary complications and stroke. However, in other patients, the disease may present with a relatively mild clinical phenotype and minimal morbidity. The cause of these differences is unclear. Possible factors that influence the severity of anemia may be inherited or non-inherited. The inherited factors include type of β-thalassemia, coinheritance of α-thalassemia, and factors that stimulate HbF production.

The dramatic advancement in the field of chelation therapy, amelioration of the clinical phenotype by genetic factors, gene therapy using lentiviral vectors, development of embryonic-like stem cells obtained by transfection, and reprogramming of differentiated somatic cells with key regulatory factors may open up a prospective generalized cure for hemoglobinopathies including thalassemia and SCD.

This book entitled *Inherited Hemoglobin Disorders* describes the genetic defects of hemoglobins, disease complications, and therapeutic strategies. This book has two distinct sections. The first theme includes seven chapters devoted to the types of hemoglobinopathies, mutation spectrum, diagnostic methods, and disease complications, and the second theme includes three chapters focusing on various treatment strategies. The content of the chapters presented in the book is guided by the knowledge and experience of the contributing authors. This book serves as an important resource and review to the researchers in the field of hemoglobinopathies.

An overview of the current hemoglobin analysis techniques and the technologies that have the potential to translate into widespread clinical settings has been presented in Chapters 1 and 2.

Chapter 3 gives an elaborate account of thalassemia, its types, mutations involved, and detection methods including the present molecular techniques. The authors of this chapter have also described as to how the modifier loci play a role in the regulation of hemoglobin synthesis.

Chapter 4 provides information on sickle cell disease, especially in Middle East Arab countries.

Chapter 5 discusses the interaction between erythropoiesis and iron overload in β-thalassemia and also gives an insight into how recent discoveries on iron metabolism and erythropoiesis could lead to new therapeutic strategies.

Chapter 6 aims to highlight the current knowledge on the epidemiology, pathophysiology, diagnosis, and treatment of acute splenic crisis associated with sickle cell disease.

Chapter 7 discusses the application of the hemoglobin release test developed by the authors to observe the re-released hemoglobin from RBCs. The re-released Hb was speculated to have a relationship with the abnormality of erythrocyte membrane and Hb.

Chapter 8 focuses on the respective contributions of known modifiers and also the pharmaceutical agents currently in use and under clinical trials for regulating the globin gene expression.

Chapter 9 discusses the role of various genetic modifiers in ameliorating the clinical phenotype. The author has also focused on the promise of therapy protocols based on the molecular basis of β-thalassemia.

Chapter 10 provides an overview of the current treatment strategies of SCD and the advances made in medicinal chemistry to find new drug targets to treat this hematological disease.

Dr. Anjana Munshi
Associate Professor and COC,
Centre for Human Genetics,
School of Health Sciences,
Central University of Punjab,
Bathinda, Punjab, India

Section 1

Hemoglobinopathies: Types, Mutations and Disease Complications

Chapter 1

Hemoglobinopathy Approach Diagnosis and Treatment Policy

Mehrdad Payandeh and Masoud Sadeghi

Additional information is available at the end of the chapter

http://dx.doi.org/10.5772/61311

Abstract

Hemoglobinopathies are the most common single gene disorders worldwide with a considerable frequency in certain area particularly Mediterranean and Middle Eastern countries. Hemoglobinopathies include structural variants of hemoglobin (Hb S, Hb C, HbE,...) and thalassaemias which are inherited defects in the globin chains synthesis. The present study was conducted to determine the prevalence of hemoglobinopathies in western Iranian patients. A total of 344 patients (151 males and 193 females) with abnormal CBC and/or hemoglobin electrophoresis were enrolled in the present study. Cellulose acetate gel electrophoresis was performed for all patients and abnormal bands were identified by citrate agar gel electrophoresis and PCR based methods. Iron deficiency anemia (IDA) was present in 156 (45.3%) individuals. Thirty four (9.8%) patients had both iron deficiency anemia and α-thalassemia trait trait, 41(11.9%) patients were with both iron deficiency anemia and minor β-thalassemia. There were 31(9%) patients with α-thalassemia trait and 5 (2.2%) patients with Hb H disease. Fifty six (16.2%) patients had minor β-thalassemia. Also, there were 10 (2.9%) individuals homozygous for hemoglobin D-Punjab and one patient with hemoglobin G (0.3%). There was one sample with hemoglobin C. Further, we found 3 patients (0.9%) with sickle cell trait and more 3 patients (0.8%) with S/ β +-thalassemia. Our results indicated that the most frequent cause of hypochromic and/or microcytic anemia in our population was IDA and the minor β-thalassemia was the second cause that needs to more attention in screening programs.

Keywords: Hemoglobinopathies, alpha- thalassemia, beta- thalassemia, anemia

1. Introduction

These two major groups, α- and β-thalassemia, are subclassified according to absent (α0 and β0) or reduced (α+ and β+) globin chain synthesis. The difference in the amount of fetal hemoglobin (HbF) that persists into adulthood affects the severity of β-thalassemia syndromes [4]. Hemoglobinopathies are the most common single gene disorders in man. There are several hundred of these disorders, but the thalassemias—alpha and beta—and the sickling disorders make up the vast majority [1]. The wide variation in the clinical manifestation of hemoglobin disorders could be attributed to the influence of various genetic modifiers and environmental factors. The heterogenous distribution of the disease and the presence of high variation in the phenotypic manifestation of a specific mutation are major problems with the development of programs for the control of the hemoglobinopathies [2] Thalassemia is one of the most common genetic diseases worldwide, with at least 60, 000 severely affected individuals born every year [3].

2. Pathophysiology

At the molecular level, the underlying cause of thalassemia is any of a number of genetic lesions that reduce or abolish the production of the globin chains of hemoglobin. The resulting chain imbalance is the key factor initiating the damage to RBC, and it is the major pathophysiological event in all forms of the thalassemia syndromes [4]. Severe IE, chronic anemia, and hypoxia also cause increased gastrointestinal (GI) tract iron absorption [5]. Repeated blood transfusions are one of the major causes of iron overload in several of these disorders, including β-thalassemia major, which is characterized by a defective β-globin gene. In addition to repeated blood transfusions and increased iron absorption, chronic hemolysis is the major cause of tissue-iron accumulation in anemic iron-overload disorders caused by hemolytic anemia [6]. Molecular studies using nucleic acid hybridization techniques and endonuclease analysis have identified loss of alpha-gene function related to gene deletion or nondeletional mutations causing hypofunctional genes and terminator codon mutations as responsible for the various alpha-thalassemia syndromes [7]. A number of reports of heterozygous *KLF1* mutations in humans either show concomitant disruption of erythropoiesis or show little effect on HbF expression, and recent studies suggest that rare variants in *KLF1* are indeed associated with elevations in HbF, but this does not appear to occur consistently or to the same extent even with similar mutations. The basis of this variation remains to be determined and will be important to better understand the mechanisms by which KLF1 acts both directly and indirectly to affect HbF expression [6]. Also, β-thalassemia major is suspected in an infant or child younger than age 2 years with the following clinical or newborn screening findings: severe microcytic anemia, mild jaundice and hepatosplenomegaly [8].

Couples and their close relatives should be evaluated for silent or atypical alpha- and beta-mutations, and if they are detected, prenatal genetic counseling for diagnostic purposes should be provided [7].

3. Clinical manifestations

Nearly 10% beta-thalassemia patients have beta-thalassemia intermedia (TI) [10]. TI is associated with a variety of serious clinical complications that require proactive and comprehensive management such as skeletal deformities and osteopenia, compensatory extramedullary hematopoiesis and tumor formation, progressive splenomegaly, a hypercoagulable state resulting in thromboembolic events and pulmonary hypertension, and increased gastrointestinal iron absorption that often results in nontransfusional iron overload and liver damage [9]. TI patients who develop progressive anemia, fatigue, and cardiopulmonary complications also require regular transfusions to maintain Hb levels <9–10 g/dL [10, 11]. Beta-thalassemia major (also called Cooley anemia, Mediterranean anemia, and von Jaksch anemia) denotes the homozygous or compound heterozygous forms of the disease, which are characterized by severe anemia (range, 1–7 g/dL of Hb), hemolysis, and massive IE [12]. Affected infants with thalassemia major fail to thrive and become progressively pale. Feeding problems, diarrhea, irritability, recurrent bouts of fever, and enlargement of the abdomen may also occur due to splenomegaly [13].

4. Strategies for TM treatment

4.1. Transfusion therapy

Early and regular blood transfusion therapy in patients with homozygous beta-thalassemia decreases the complications of severe anemia and prolongs survival that in the long term. The beneficial effects of transfusions are limited by the organ damage resulting from iron overload, a consequence of the body's limited capacity to excrete iron, and by the complications of infection with blood-borne agents [14]. Current therapeutic approaches for homozygous beta-thalassemia entail blood transfusions and iron chelation therapy with deferoxamine or deferiprone for preventing tissue hemosiderosis. Nowadays, much effort has focused on various inducers of HbF, such as recombinant human erythropoietin, especially in beta-thalassemia intermedia [15]. Cytomegalovirus-negative blood products are recommended for potential candidates for curative stem cell transplantation (SCT). Parents and first-degree relatives should not be blood donors for these candidates. Hepatitis B vaccination is given before transfusion therapy [16]. Transfusions of washed, leukocyte-depleted RBCs are recommended for all the patients to reduce the incidence of febrile and urticarial reactions as well as infectious cytomegalovirus contamination. If they are not available, frozen–thawed RBCs should be administered [17, 18]. Current transfusion regimen guidelines state that the pretransfusion hemoglobin (Hb) should ideally be in the 9- to 10-g/dL range. This recommended transfusion scheme generally leads to the transfusion of 100–200 mL/kg/year of packed red blood cells, which is equivalent to 0.3–0.6 mg of iron per kg body weight per day [19].

4.2. Managing of the complications

Cardiac failure and serious arrhythmias are the major causes of life-threatening morbidity and mortality in iron-overload patients [20]. In the modern era, with iron chelation treatment, the clinical manifestation of cardiac disease has changed, and pericarditis and myocarditis are now rare. Historical postmortem studies showed severe replacement cardiac fibrosis [21], but this is now rare in more modern cohorts of patients dying of HF [22]. Patients receiving regular transfusion and iron chelation should be assessed formally for their cardiac status (history, physical examination, and auscultation) beginning at the age of 10 years and annually thereafter [23]. There are ongoing clinical trials that are relevant to the treatment of cardiac iron overload by deferasirox. One that is relevant is the Novartis 2214 trial, with open-label treatment in TM patients with combined deferoxamine with deferasirox. In addition, clinical trials of new chelators are ongoing [24]. Diuretics, including loop diuretics (furosemide) and potassium-sparing agents (spironolactone), as well as angiotensin-converting enzyme (ACE) inhibitors should be prescribed based on arterial blood pressure. Also, in cases of persistent normal sinus tachycardia, small doses of carvedilol and digoxin may be given and must be prescribed to patients with atrial fibrillation resistant to conversion [25].

4.3. Bone disease

Therefore, the detection of low bone mass in many regularly transfused and well-chelated β TM patients over the last decade was quite unexpected [26]. DiStefano et al. [27] reported that the etiology of bone disease in thalassemia is poorly understood. Therefore, a number of studies have examined the effect of various conditions on the pathogenesis of bone disease, including ineffective erythropoiesis, iron overload, treatment with DFO, vitamin D concentrations, influence of endocrinopathies (such as hypogonadism and growth hormone deficiency), and thalassemia genotype. Beginning in childhood, yearly examination of bone mineral density as well as calcium, vitamin D3 metabolism, and thyroid and parathyroid functions should be performed. Some short-term success has been seen with the administration of pamidronate in patients with Z-/T-score <2.5. It seems that early administration of iron chelation is effective in preventing endocrine complications [28].

4.4. Splenectomy

Splenectomy determines immediate drop in blood consumption and iron intake but slow downtrend of ferritin, which are direct measurements of iron overload [29]. Also, Splenectomy reduces transfusion requirements in the first year after surgery in patients with thalassemia major and hypersplenism [30]. Splenectomy should generally be avoided in NTDT patients <5 years, and it should be reserved for the following cases [31]:

a. When transfusion therapy is not possible or iron chelation therapy is unavailable

b. Worsening anemia leading to poor growth and development

c. Hypersplenism and splenomegaly

d. Leading to worsening anemia, leucopenia, or thrombocytopenia and causing clinical problems such as recurrent bacterial infections or bleeding

e. Accompanied by symptoms such as left upper quadrant pain or early satiety

f. Massive splenomegaly (>20 cm) with concern about possible splenic rupture

The susceptibility to overwhelming infections after splenectomy can be reduced by immunization with pneumococcal and meningococcal vaccines before splenectomy and antimicrobial prophylaxis with penicillin after splenectomy [32]. In cases of ongoing transfusion therapy, with each RBC unit containing >200 mg of iron, cumulative iron burden is an inevitable consequence [33].

4.5. Prevention: prenatal diagnosis

The prenatal diagnosis of β-thalassemia was accomplished for the first time in the 1970s by globin chain synthesis analysis on fetal blood obtained by placental aspiration at 18–22 weeks gestation [34]. Acceptance of prenatal diagnosis and termination of affected fetuses are dependent on the early identification of couples at risk, culturally sensitive genetic counseling, cost, and religious beliefs even when PCR technologies are available [35]. Preimplantation genetic diagnosis is generally defined as the testing of preimplantation stage embryos or oocytes for genetic defects, and preimplantation embryo diagnosis requires in vitro fertilization, embryo biopsy, and using either fluorescent in situ hybridization or polymerase chain reaction at the single cell level [36]. Current PCR technologies and precise hybridization assays to detect single point mutations with great reliability using very small DNA samples have been developed. New technology using fetal DNA obtained from maternal plasma or maternal peripheral blood has also been developed but is not routinely available [37].

4.6. Cure: HSCT

Hematopoietic SCT (HSCT) is an established procedure for many acquired and congenital disorders of the hematopoietic system [38]. The European Group for Bone Marrow Transplantation analyses in previous years have shown an increase in the annual absolute HSCT numbers and transplant rates (number of HSCT/10 million inhabitants) of about 4–13% (median 8%) for allogeneic and 1.5–9.5% (median 4%) for autologous HSCT [39]. The success of an allogeneic HSCT is dependent on a multitude of factors, including the procurement of an optimal graft source. Further, the quality of this graft depends on a variety of donor and/or host characteristics. Most importantly, HLA compatibility between the recipient and the donor is considered the dominant characteristic in this field [40]. There are other important donor characteristics that these non-HLA characteristics may be broadly considered to be either traditional characteristics, such as ABO compatibility or novel, such as cytokine or KIR polymorphisms [41]. Approximately 10% of SCT patients are transfusion-free for years, although they experience persistent mixed hematopoietic chimerism [42]. This suggests that only a few engrafted donor cells are sufficient for correction of donor phenotype. Approximately 30% subsequently reject their grafts. Another option is to use matched unrelated donor if a matched sibling is not available or when patients are not compliant with conventional therapy [43].

4.7. Cord blood transplantation

Although the clinical application of hematopoietic cell transplantation has relied on marrow collected from related and unrelated donors as the primary source of donor hematopoietic cells, umbilical cord blood (UCB) is an alternative source of hematopoietic cells and represents a suitable allogeneic donor pool in the event that a marrow donor is not available [44]. The small size or small number of stem cells in the UBC collection relative to the number required for engraftment are probably the main causes of failure of UCB transplantation; therefore, this procedure is being used mainly in pediatric patients [45].

5. Therapies for future

5.1. Fetal hemoglobin inducers

Recently, a novel therapeutic strategy (HbF) has been hypothesized for β-thalassemia, based on the observation that the coexistence of the hereditary persistence of fetal hemoglobin in patients with β-thalassemia reduces the severity of the disease [46]. Several drugs, including erythropoietin, demethylating agents, such as 5-azacytidine, and short chain fatty acids, such as butyrate, have been studied individually and in various combinations [7]. Hydroxyurea (HU), which is very effective in increasing HbF levels, has been used extensively for many years in patients with sickle cell anemia (SCA) [47].

5.2. Gene therapy

Requirements for effective gene transfer for the treatment of β-thalassemia are regulated, erythroid-specific, consistent, and high-level β-globin or γ-globin expression that Gamma retroviral vectors have had great success with immune deficiency disorders, but due to vector-associated limitations, they have limited utility in hemoglobinopathies. Nowadays, lentivirus vectors have been shown in several studies to correct mouse and animal models of thalassemia [48]. In total, concerns regarding gene transfer include the need for improved efficiency of gene delivery and mastery of vector stability, viral titers, nononcogenic insertion, the variable expression of globin genes, and the variable contributions of the beta-thalassemia phenotype and other modifiers to the effectiveness of gene transfer [49].

Author details

Mehrdad Payandeh* and Masoud Sadeghi

*Address all correspondence to: md.payandeh@yahoo.com

Department of Hematology, Medical Oncology and Bone Marrow Transplantation, Kermanshah University of Medical Sciences, Kermanshah, Iran

References

[1] Sarnaik SA. Thalassemia and related hemoglobinopathies. Indian J Pediatr. 2005 Apr; 72(4):319–24.

[2] Rahimi Z. Genetic epidemiology, hematological and clinical features of hemoglobinopathies in Iran. Biomed Res Int. 2013;2013:803487.

[3] Higgs DR, Engel JD, Stamatoyannopoulos G. Thalassaemia. Lancet. 2012 Jan 28;379(9813):373–83.

[4] Rund D, Rachmilewitz E. Pathophysiology of alpha- and beta-thalassemia: therapeutic implications. Semin Hematol. 2001 Oct;38(4):343–9.

[5] Schwartz E Jr. Thalassemia syndromes. In: Miller D, Baehner R, eds. Smith's Blood Diseases of Infancy and Childhood (6th ed.). St. Louis, MO: Mosby; 1989:428.

[6] Anderson ER, Taylor M, Xue X, Ramakrishnan SK, Martin A, Xie L, et al. Intestinal HIF2α promotes tissue-iron accumulation in disorders of iron overload with anemia. Proc Natl Acad Sci U S A. 2013 Dec 10;110(50):E4922–30.

[7] Giardina P, Forget B. Thalassemia syndromes. In: Hoffman R, Benz E, Shattil S, et al., eds. Hematology: Basic Principles and Practice (5th ed.). Philadelphia, PA: Churchill Livingstone; 2008:535–63.

[8] Pagon RA, Bird TC, Dolan CR, Stephens K, Cao A, Galanello R In: Pagon RA, Bird TC, Dolan CR, Stephens K, eds. GeneReviews [Internet] Beta-Thalassemia. Seattle, WA: University of Washington, Seattle; 1993–2000 [updated 2010].

[9] Taher AT, Musallam KM, Karimi M, Cappellini MD. Contemporary approaches to treatment of beta-thalassemia intermedia. Blood Rev. 2012 Apr;26 Suppl 1:S24–7.

[10] Aessopos A, Farmakis D, Karagiorga M, et al. Cardiac involvement in thalassemia intermedia: a multicenter study. Blood. 2001;97(11):3411–6.

[11] Aessopos A, Farmakis D, Deftereos S, et al. Thalassemia heart disease: a comparative evaluation of thalassemia major and thalassemia intermedia. Chest. 2005;127(5):1523–30.

[12] Schwartz E Jr. Thalassemia syndromes. In: Miller D, Baehner R, eds. Smith's Blood Diseases of Infancy and Childhood (6th ed.). St. Louis, MO: Mosby; 1989:428.

[13] Cao A, Galanello R. Beta-thalassemia. Genet Med. 2010 Feb;12(2):61–76.

[14] Prati D. Benefits and complications of regular blood transfusion in patients with beta-thalassaemia major. Vox Sang. 2000;79(3):129–37.

[15] Chaidos A, Makis A, Hatzimichael E, Tsiara S, Gouva M, Tzouvara E, et al. Treatment of beta-thalassemia patients with recombinant human erythropoietin: effect on transfusion requirements and soluble adhesion molecules. Acta Haematol. 2004;111(4):189–95.

[16] Di Marco V, Capra M, Angelucci E, et al. Manage- ment of chronic viral hepatitis in patients with thalassemia: recommendations from an international panel. Blood. 2010;116(16):2875–83.

[17] Piomelli S, Graziano J, Karpatkin M, et al. Chelation therapy, transfusion requirement, and iron balance in young thalassemic patients. Ann N Y Acad Sci. 1980;344:409–417.

[18] Piomelli S, Hart D, Graziano J, et al. Current strategies in the management of Cooley's anemia. Ann N Y Acad Sci. 1985;445:256–67.

[19] Cazzola M, De Stefano P, Ponchio L, Locatelli F, Beguin Y, Dessi C, et al. Relationship between transfusion regimen and suppression of erythropoiesis in beta-thalassaemia major. Br J Haematol. 1995;89:473–8.

[20] Modell B, Khan M, Darlison M. Survival in beta-thalassaemia major in the UK: data from the UK Thalassaemia Register. Lancet. 2000;355(9220): 2051–2.

[21] Buja LM, Roberts WC. Iron in the heart: etiology and clinical significance. Am J Med. 1971;51:209–21.

[22] Kirk P, Sheppard M, Carpenter J, Anderson L, He T, De Noronha S, et al. Fibrosis in cardiac siderosis: update on historical perspectives. Haematologica. 2012;97 (e-Suppl 1):382.

[23] Pennell DJ, Udelson JE, Arai AE, Bozkurt B, Cohen AR, Galanello R, et al. Cardiovascular function and treatment in β-thalassemia major: a consensus statement from the American Heart Association. Circulation. 2013 Jul 16;128(3):281–308.

[24] Jensen JH, Tang H, Tosti CL, Swaminathan SV, Nunez A, Hultman K, et al. Separate MRI quantification of dispersed (ferritin-like) and aggregated (hemosiderin-like) storage iron. Magn Reson Med. 2010;63:1201–9.

[25] Aessopos A, Berdoukas V, Tsironi M. The heart in transfusion dependent homozygous thalassaemia today – prediction, prevention and management. Eur J Haematol. 2008 Feb;80(2):93–106. Epub 2007 Dec 10.

[26] Jensen CE, Tuck SM, Agnew JE, Koneru S, Morris RW, Yardumian A, et al. High incidence of osteoporosis in thalassemia major. J Pediatr Endocrinol Metab. 1998;11(Suppl 3):975–977.

[27] DiStefano M, Chiabotto P, Roggia C, Garofalo F, Lala R, Piga A, et al. Bone mass and metabolism in thalassemic children and adolescents with different iron cheating drugs. J Bone Miner Metab. 2004;22:53–57.

[28] Cunningham MJ, Macklin EA, Neufeld EJ, Cohen AR. Complications of beta-thalassemia major in North America. Blood. 2004;104(1):34- 39.

[29] Casale M, Cinque P, Ricchi P, Costantini S, Spasiano A, Prossomariti L, et al. Effect of splenectomy on iron balance in patients with β-thalassemia major: a long-term follow-up. Eur J Haematol. 2013 Jul;91(1):69–73.

[30] Cohen A, Gayer R, Mizanin J. Long-term effect of splenectomy on transfusion requirements in thalassemia major. Am J Hematol. 1989 Apr;30(4):254–6.

[31] Taher A, Vichinsky E, Musallam K, Cappellini MD, Viprakasit V. Guidelines for the Management of Non Tranfusion Dependent Thalassemia (NTDT). Cyprus: Thalassemia International Federation; 2013.

[32] Ikeda M, Sekimoto M, Takiguchi S, et al. High incidence of thrombosis of the portal venous system after laparoscopic splenectomy: a prospective study with contrast-enhanced CT scan. Ann Surg. 2005;241(2):208–16.

[33] Pippard M. Iron chelation therapy in the treatment of iron overload. In: Bergeron R, Brittenham G, eds. The Development of Iron Chelators for Clinical Use. Boca Raton, FL: CRC Press; 1994:57–74.

[34] Rosetalli M, Saba L. Prenatal diagnosis of β-thalassemias and hemoglobinopathies. Mediterr J Hematol Infect Dis. 2009; 1(1): e2009011.

[35] Petrou M. Preimplantation genetic diagnosis. Hemoglobin. 2009;33(Suppl 1):S7–13.

[36] Geraedts JP, De Wert GM. Preimplantation genetic diagnosis. Clin Genet. 2009 Oct; 76(4):315–25.

[37] Chiu RW, Lau TK, Leung TN, Chow KC, Chui DH, Lo YM. Prenatal exclusion of beta thalassaemia major by examination of maternal plasma. Lancet. 2002;360(9338):998–1000.

[38] Gratwohl A, Baldomero H, Aljurf M, Pasquini MC, Bouzas LF, Yoshimi A, et al. Hematopoietic stem cell transplantation: a global perspective. JAMA. 2010;303:1617–24.

[39] Passweg JR, Baldomero H, Bregni M, Cesaro S, Dreger P, Duarte RF, et al. Hematopoietic SCT in Europe: data and trends in 2011. Bone Marrow Transplant. 2013 Sep; 48(9):1161–7.

[40] Flomenberg N, Baxter-Lowe LA, Confer D, Fernandez-Vina M, Filipovich A, Horowitz M, et al. Impact of HLA class I and class II high-resolution matching on outcomes of unrelated donor bone marrow transplantation: HLA-C mismatching is associated with a strong adverse effect on transplantation outcome. Blood 2004; 104: 1923–30.

[41] Drummond MF, Sculpher MJ, Torrance GW, O'Brien BJ, Stoddart GL. Methods for Economic Evaluation of Health Care Programmes. Oxford University Press, Oxford; 2005, p 234.

[42] Cappellini MD, Cohen A, Piga A, Bejaoui M, Perrotta S, Agaoglu L, et al. A phase 3 study of deferasirox (ICL670), a once-daily oral iron chelator, in patients with beta-thalassemia. Blood. 2006 May 1;107(9):3455–62.

[43] Gaziev J, Sodani P, Polchi P, et al. Bone marrow transplantation in adults with thalassemia: treatment and long-term follow-up. Ann N Y Acad Sci. 2005;1054:196–205.

[44] Kanathezhath B, Walters MC. Umbilical cord blood transplantation for thalassemia major. 2010 Dec;24(6):1165–77.

[45] Boncimino A, Bertaina A, Locatelli F. Cord blood transplantation in patients with hemoglobinopathies. Transfus Apher Sci. 2010;42(3):277–81.

[46] Gambari R. Foetal haemoglobin inducers and thalassaemia: novel achievements. Blood Transfus. 2010 Jan;8(1):5–7.

[47] Dixit A, Chatterjee TC, Mishra P, et al. Hydroxyurea in thalassemia intermedia: a promising therapy. Ann Hematol. 2005;84(7):441–6.

[48] Arumugam P, Malik P. Genetic therapy for beta-thalassemia: from the bench to the bedside. Hematology Am Soc Hematol Educ Program. 2010;2010:445–50.

[49] Rivella S, Rachmilewitz E. Future alternative therapies for beta-thalassemia. Expert Rev He matol. 2009;2(6):685.

Chapter 2

Thalassemia — From Genotype to Phenotype

Ghada Y. El-Kamah and Khalda S. Amr

Additional information is available at the end of the chapter

http://dx.doi.org/10.5772/61433

Abstract

Thalassemia encompasses serious diseases with complex pathophysiology that is difficult to explain since it is considered a group of defects with similar clinical effects, still not a single disorder.

Understanding genetic factors contributing to the pathophysiology of thalassemias has enabled the identification of causative genes and development of diagnostic tests, helping defuse the confusion that evolves from clinical descriptions alone and correlating clinical symptoms with thalassemia disease.

More than 300 disease-causing mutations have been identified so far, mostly behaving as Mendelian recessives, however, there are variants that cause a disease phenotype even when present in a single copy. The remarkable technical developments of molecular biology gradually make it possible to define many of the globin gene molecular underlying pathologies.

Still, current morbidity and mortality remain unacceptable underlining the need for further research in this area.

In this chapter, we have summarized the current state of knowledge in the field of molecular lesions that underlie thalassemias, how they relate to their phenotypes, as well as the importance of conveying to the reader the extent to which it is possible to explain their clinical heterogeneity at the molecular level.

Keywords: Thalassemias, genotype/phenotype correlation, molecular heterogeneity

1. Introduction

During the past few years there has been a rapid increase of knowledge in the field of genetic control of hemoglobin synthesis in health and disease, which led to reviving the interest in thalassemia and associated disorders of hemoglobin (Hb) production.

Interest in the Hb molecule arose from its changes in a series of common clinical intermingled conditions, caused either by its structural variants (hemoglobinopathies), defects of synthesis (thalassemias), or a diverse group of defects in the developmental progression from fetal to adult hemoglobin production (HPFH) [1].

The revelation of the molecular basis of thalassemia lead to the concept of "molecular pathology and molecular medicine", with a shift of *emphasis* from illness in patients or their organs to pathological affection at the cellular and molecular level. Furthermore the study of these disorders shows great promise of answering some fundamental questions about the genetic mechanisms involved in defective protein synthesis [2].

Thalassemias are a group of inherited microcytic, hemolytic anemias characterized by defective Hb synthesis. It is now clear that thalassemias occur much more frequently, and in more racial groups, than was previously realized. Thalassemias confer a degree of protection against malaria, due to the blood cells' easy degradation. This selective survival advantage of carriers or heterozygous advantage may be responsible for the perpetuation of the mutation in some populations [3].

Generally, thalassemias affect all races, particularly people of Mediterranean origin, Arabs, and Asians with variable incidences, where the highest reported rate is in the Maldives (18% carriers' rate), followed by that of descendants from Latin American and Mediterranean countries while the reported incidence rate is very low in Northern Europe (0.1%) and Africa (0.9%) [3,4].

Acquired abnormalities of hemoglobin synthesis may also arise as a secondary manifestation of hematologic neoplasia and can be seen in any population. However, it is more readily recognized where inherited hemoglobin abnormalities are rare and less likely to cause diagnostic confusion [5].

This high prevalence of thalassemia makes it one of the major health problems and a priority genetic disease. Treatment of β-thalassemia, albeit more and more available, still represents a significant drain of the country's resources due to the disease's major complications. A prevention program would be useful to overcome these problems, but it requires a preliminary knowledge of hemoglobin, disease pathophysiology, as well as a spectrum of globin gene mutations among different populations [6].

2. Pathophysiology

Thalassemias are caused either by variant or missing genes affecting hemoglobin (Hb) production.

Human hemoglobin is formed of four peptide (globin) chains, and these chains are differentially produced during ontogeny; hence, they are diverse at the embryonic, fetal, and adult stages [1].

http://dx.doi.org/10.5772/61433

Reviewing the genesis of the normal post-embryonal hemoglobins can facilitate understanding thalassemias.

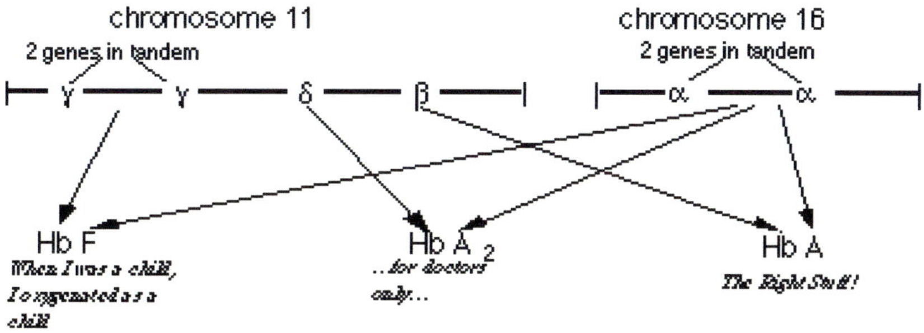

Figure 1. Normal adult human hemoglobins [7]

During embryonic development, zeta and epsilon (ζ &ε) globin chains disappear at 8 weeks to be replaced by α chains. In fetal life, Hb F ($\alpha2\gamma2$) is the predominant Hb. The whole Hb transition is completed by 6 months of postnatal life, with 97% Hb A ($\alpha2\beta2$), 3% or less Hb A2 ($\alpha2\delta2$), and up to 1% Hb F (Fig. 1) in a normal adult [8]. These transitions among different hemoglobins are a reflection of the physiological adaptions to differing oxygen requirements at various stages of development.

The normal adult's Hb molecule is a spheroidal protein that contains two pairs of different globin molecules. It consists of four protein subunits arranged like a thick-walled shell with a central cavity forming an ellipsoidal tetrahedron (Fig. 2).

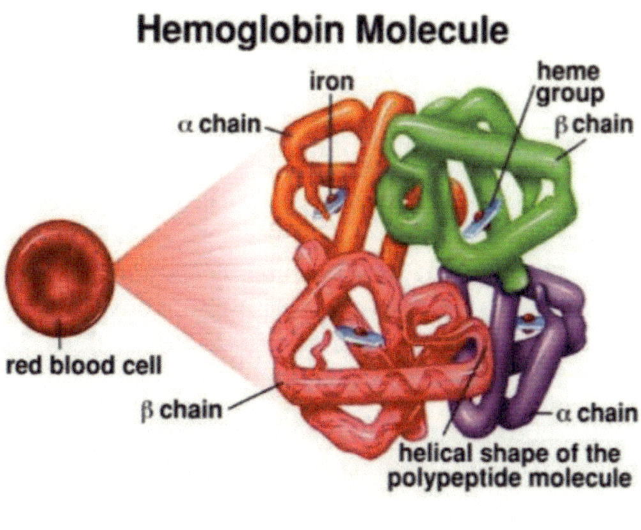

Figure 2. The structure of hemoglobin (Hb) [10]

The four subunits are two pairs of identical polypeptide chains: a pair of identical α or α-like chains and a pair of identical non-α or non-α-like chains. Each chain is associated with one haem molecule on the interior of the shell that is essential for oxygen uptake and release. The two α-like chains contain 141 amino acids while the non-α-like chains contain 146 amino acids [9].

The structure of globin genes has been highly conserved throughout evolution. Their transcribed regions are contained in three exons, separated by two introns. From the CAP site, the start of transcription, the first exon encompasses ~50 bp of 5′ untranslated sequence (UTR) in which a TATA, CAAT, and duplicated CACCC boxes and a major regulatory region, containing a strong enhancer, maps 50 Kb from the beta globin gene.

Exon 1 encodes also codons for amino acids 1–31 in the **α**- and 1–29 in addition to the first two bases of codon 30 in the β-globin genes [9]. While exon 2 encodes amino acids 32–99 in the **α**- and 31–104 in the β-globin genes, that is the portion of the globin polypeptide involved in haem binding and the **α**1β2 (**α**2β1) contacts. The remaining amino acids (100–141 for **α**, 105–146 for β), together with a 3′ untranslated region of ~100 bp, are encoded in exon three [9] (Fig. 3).

In **α**-globin genes both introns are small, 117–149bp. The first intervening sequence in β-like genes is also small, 122–130bp, while IVS2 is much larger, 850–904bp. The removal of the intervening sequences from the initial transcript and joining the exon sequence to form mRNA is dependent on consensus sequences of exon-intron boundaries. At the 5′ end of each intron the consensus is CAAG/GTAGAGT, where the excision site immediately precedes the invariant GT residues, the splice donor site. At the 3′ end, the acceptor site, an invariant AG dinucleotide within a looser consensus (CT)N CT AG/G precedes the excision site and terminates the codon [9]. These consensus sequences are strongly upheld and in all cases GT and AG dinucleotides are maintained. As mutations in these sequences frequently lead to thalassemia, the globin genes provide excellent examples of their functional importance [9].

The expression and regulation of globin genes depend on the interactions of different trans-acting regulatory promoters, a series of enhancing elements and a "master" regulatory region involved in regulating the entire **α**- or β-globin gene complex. Widely expressed "housekeeping" genes that lack tissue specificity and maintain an early replicating, open chromatin structure in both erythroid and non-erythroid cells surround the α cluster. There are several upstream DNase1 hypersensitive sites (HSs), four of which are erythroid specific. Only one of these sites, 40kb upstream from the ζ globin gene, has strong enhancer activity (HS-40); this site is believed to be the major α globin gene regulatory element. It lies in an intron of a neighboring widely expressed gene (C16orf35) of unknown function. Knowledge of interactions of these sequences with both erythroid-specific and more generally active regulatory proteins is continuously acquired, however, details about how these complex interactions underlie the control of the globin-gene clusters remain to be worked out [9].

Ultimately, a very tightly controlled globin chain production process keeps the ratio of α- chains to non-α- chains, at 1.00 (± 0.05). Thalassemia, by altering this process, disrupts this ratio [11].

The basic pathology in all forms of thalassemia is a result of the presence of excess unstable globin chains within the affected RBCs. The effects of unstable hemoglobin chains on the

RBC membrane components are not the same and the pattern and rate of their precipitation differs [12].

Unlike the surfeit of α-chains that is produced in β-thalassemia, excess γ and β chains that result from defective α-chain production are able to form soluble homo tetramers, γ4 (or Hb Bart's) and β4 (or Hb H), which are physiologically useless because of their very high oxygen affinity as well as their instability in case of Hb H [9]. The clinical features of the more severe forms of α-thalassemia are therefore considered a reflection of hemoglobin Bart's and H properties as well as their effects on erythropoiesis, particularly on red-cell survival [9,13].

The unbalanced Hb synthesis, which is the principle of the pathophysiology of thalassemia, is caused by decreased production of at least one of the major globin polypeptide chains: alpha (α), beta (β), gamma (γ), delta (δ), and *epsilon (ε).*

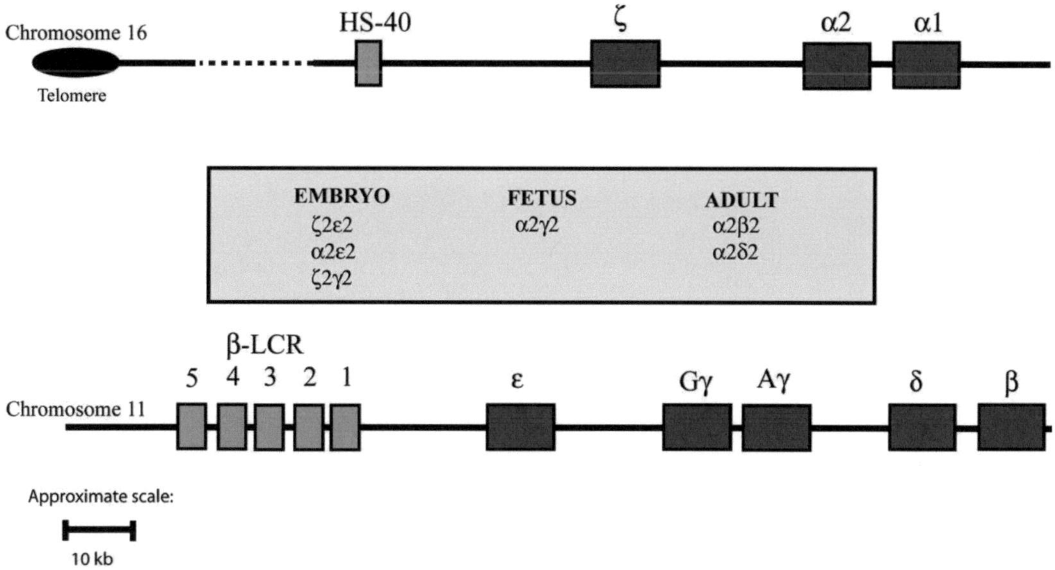

Figure 3. Schematic representation of the human globin gene clusters. ζ, α2, and α1 globin genes situated near the telomeric region of the short arm of chromosome 16. About 40 kb upstream of the 5′ end of the ζ globin gene is the HS-40 α-globin genes remote regulatory region. The β-like globin cluster is located on the short arm of chromosome 11; upstream of the cluster is the β-globin gene remote regulatory locus control region (β-LCR). In between are represented the different ontogenetic stages of Hb [14]

3. Different types of thalassemia

- **α-Thalassemia** results from decreased alpha globin chain production. It is most commonly inherited as a recessive Mendelian disorder. Acquired α-thalassemia was reported under rare circumstances [14]. The production of α-globin chains is directed by two functional alpha genes (α1 and α2) located in the α-globin gene cluster at the short arm of chromosome 16p13.3 [15], which comprises two ψα- genes followed by two α-globin genes [Fig. 4] in the same order as their expression throughout development [16].

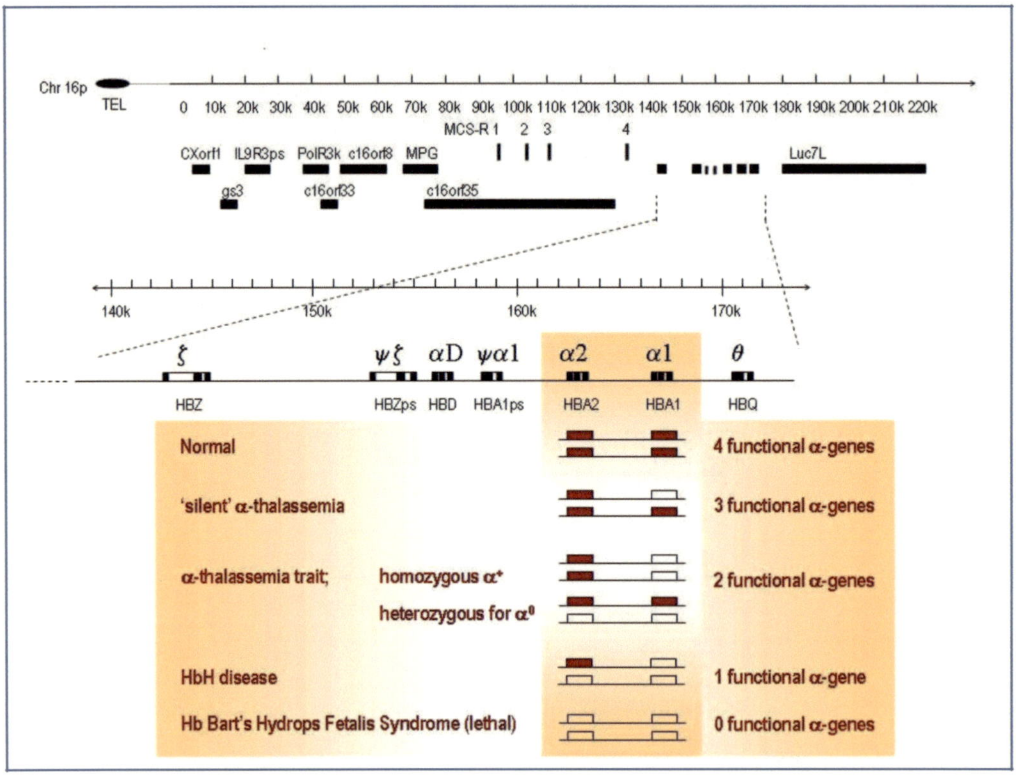

Figure 4. α-globin gene cluster on chromosome 16. The telomere is shown as an oval, genes are shown as boxes, and α-globin regulatory region (MCS-R 1 to 4) is indicated as vertical bars. The genotype/phenotype relationship is shown in the entailed table [17]

Decreased production of alpha2-globin or alpha1-globin gene products yields a relative excess of beta chains, which results in less stable chains with consequent clinical disease [18,19].

The severity of α thalassemias is correlated with the α globin genes affection; deletional or nondeletional mutations involving one (α+) or both (α°) alpha genes *in cis* at the α gene cluster resulting in four clinical phenotypes of α-thalassemia. The silent carrier state is caused by heterozygosity to the α+ defect. However, α-thalassemia minor is caused by either homozygosity to the α+ defects or heterozygosity to the α° defects [20].

Defects in 3 of the 4 genes severely impair α-chain production, resulting in tetramers of excess β chains (Hb H) or, in infancy, γ chains (Bart's Hb). Defects in all 4 genes are a lethal condition in utero as the lack of α chains affects O_2 transport [19].

- **β-Thalassemia** results from decreased production of β-polypeptide chains (β^+), or β^0 where no beta globin is produced. A less severe form β^{++} thalassemia denotes mild defect in β-chain production [21].

β-globin is encoded by a structural gene found in a cluster with other α-like genes spanning 70 Kb on the short arm of chromosome 11 (11p15.4) (Fig. 3). Beta thalassemia inheritance is autosomal recessive: Heterozygotes are carriers and have asymptomatic mild to moderate microcytic anemia (thalassemia minor); homozygotes develop variable phenotypes, ranging from the severe transfusion dependent thalassemia major to the mild form of thalassemia intermedia [21]. The diagnostic feature of β-thalassemia is an elevated level of HbA2 in heterozygotes, found in most forms of β^0 and β^+ thalassemia. However, there are less common cases of normal HbA2 β-thalassemia with normal HbA2 level in heterozygotes [9].

- **δ-thalassemia** – about 3% of adult hemoglobin is made of α and δ chains. Mutations affecting δ-globin gene produce δ^0 or δ^+ thalassemia [22]. Mutations in the δ-globin gene are not pathologically relevant [23]. However, since high HbA2 levels are diagnostic for beta-thalassemia trait, co-inheritance of δ- and β- gene defects or **β-δ-thalassemia** may lead to misinterpretation of diagnostic results through preventing an elevation of the level of HbA2 [23].
- **HPFH** is characterized by persistent fetal hemoglobin synthesis in adult life in the absence of major hematological abnormalities. HPFH can modify the clinical phenotype of the β-thalassemia and reduce their severity. Many forms of HPFH are considered as extremely well compensated forms of β- or δβ-thalassemia [23,24]. In some forms there is no δ or β chain production and almost complete compensation by a high output of γ chains **$(\delta\beta)^0$ HPFH**. In other forms, the β- and δ-chain synthesis cis are directed by genes on the same chromosome, to the HPFH determinant, hence designated $^G\gamma\beta^+$ or $^A\gamma\beta^+$ HPFH, depending on the structure of the Hb F [9].

Another heterogeneous group of HPFH is present in otherwise normal individuals with much lower levels of Hb F. Evidence is mounting that the genetic determinants for some types of this form of HPFH are not linked to the β-globin gene cluster [9].

- **εγδβ-Thalassemia** is a rare disease that results from loss of either the whole or a major part of the β-like globin-gene cluster and its regulatory regions. Strictly speaking, therefore, it should be described as $(\varepsilon^G\gamma^A\gamma\delta\beta)^0$ thalassemia. Homozygotes would not be compatible with life; heterozygotes have the clinical phenotype of β-thalassemia with a normal HbA2 level [9].
- **γ-Thalassemia** is not associated with imbalanced globin production and hence does not appear to be of clinical significance. Deletions involving one or more of the γ-globin genes have only been identified during surveys of the relative levels of $^G\gamma$ and $^A\gamma$ chains in Hb F. Only one form of γ-thalassemia has been described due to about 5 Kb deletion at the 3′ end of the $^G\gamma$ gene, the 5′ end of the $^A\gamma$ gene and the intergenic region. Most likely it resulted from unequal cross overs between $^G\gamma$ and $^A\gamma$ resulting in - $^{GA}\gamma$-hybrid gene [2,25].
- **Thalassemia due to inheritance of structural Hb variant**

Hemoglobin E/thalassemia: Common in India, Bangladesh, and throughout Southeast Asia and although previously rarely diagnosed in North America or Europe, it has become the most common form of β-thalassemia detected through many newborn screening programs. It is clinically characterized by marked variability, ranging from mild asymptomatic anemia to a life-threatening disorder requiring transfusions from infancy [2,26].

Hemoglobin S/thalassemia is common in African and Mediterranean populations. Coinheritance of α or β-globin gene mutations can modulate the hematological diagnostic data and clinical expression of the sickle cell. The phenotype of the β-globin gene defect determines the severity of the co-inherited sickle cell mutation; β^0 results in a severe disease, while β^+ causes a milder clinical picture of the disease [27]. Its coexistence with α-thalassemia (α^{thal}) lowers MCV& MCH, resulting in milder anemia, but causes a reduction in hemolysis and increase in total hemoglobin, which makes patients more prone to vaso-occlusive and painful crises [28].

Hemoglobin C/thalassemia is common in Mediterranean and African populations. HB C usually results in mild asymptomatic anemia; however, hemoglobin C/β^o thalassemia can cause moderately severe hemolytic anemia with splenomegaly while hemoglobin C/β^+ thalassemia produces a milder disease [29].

Hemoglobin D/thalassemia is common in the northwestern parts of India and Pakistan (Punjab region). Hb D homozygotes are asymptomatic. Coinheritance of Hb D/β-thalassemia results in mild anemia ± mild splenomegaly while coinheritance with α-thalassemia results in higher Hb levels [30].

4. Molecular pathology/relevance to phenotype

Thalassemia is a difficult disease to explain, since it is considered a group of defects with similar clinical effects, still not a single disorder.

Molecular characterization of thalassemia is of great importance in helping defuse the confusion that evolves from clinical descriptions alone. Therefore, the best approach is to understand the genetic background in correlation with clinical symptoms of patients with thalassemia disease.

The remarkable technical developments of molecular biology gradually make it possible to define many of the globin gene molecular underlying pathologies. Herein we will try to summarize the molecular lesions that underlie thalassemias, how they relate to their phenotypes, as well as the importance of conveying to the reader the extent to which it is possible to explain their clinical heterogeneity at the molecular level.

The molecular basis of the thalassemias has been scrupulously expounded and represents one of the first diseases to be characterized at the molecular level.

Different mutations; point mutations, small insertions, deletions, or, in some cases, partial or large deletions encompassing one or two globin genes alter the function of the genes encoding a globin chain [31].

For example, mutations resulting in the absence of β-chain synthesis (β^0-thalassemia) are at times caused by β-globin gene deletions or more commonly by subtle mutations such as nonsense, frame shift, or RNA-splicing mutations [31]. While in β^+ thalassemia with only reduction in β chain synthesis, β-globin gene mutations may be located in promoter regions, at exon-intron boundaries disrupting splice site recognition, within introns generating cryptic splice signals or farther downstream at sites that regulate RNA stability [31].

On the other hand, non-deletional α-thalassemia mutations are not as prevalent as the deletional mutations. However, they were reported in some regions with high consanguinity rates such as in Saudi Arabia and the surrounding Gulf countries [31]. Deletion mutations affecting one, two, or three α-globin genes yield mild to severe hemolytic anemia. Deletion of all four α-globin genes results in homozygous α-thalassemia clinically manifesting as hydrops fetalis, a condition associated with stillbirth [31].

Genetic classification of α-thalassemia

Analysis of the human α-globin cluster has revealed a remarkable degree of structural variability due to point mutations, deletions, and insertions of DNA.

The α-globin genes are embedded within two highly homologous 4 kb duplication units, the sequence identity of which has been maintained throughout evolution by gene conversion and unequal crossover events [9]. These regions are divided into homologous sub-segments (X, Y, and Z). α-thalassemia is classified according to its cause into deletional and non-deletional as follows.

α^+-thalassemia due to deletions ; α-thalassemia is more frequently caused by deletion. One of the most common α-thalassemia deletions is the rightward deletion due to reciprocal recombination between Z segments that are 3.7 kb apart, producing a chromosome with only one α-globin gene (–α3.7, rightward deletion) causing α-thalassemia and α-triplication allele without a thalassemic effect (Fig. 5).

Another common crossover between homologous X boxes, which are 4.2 kb apart, also gives rise to an α-thalassemia determinant (–α 4.2) and an α-triplication allele anti4.2 chromosome [32]. Further recombination events could give rise to other unusual rearrangements. Other rare deletions that produce α+ thalassemia have also been described, for example, deletion of the entire α-1 gene and its flanking DNA (–α3.5) [Fig. 6] [9, 33].

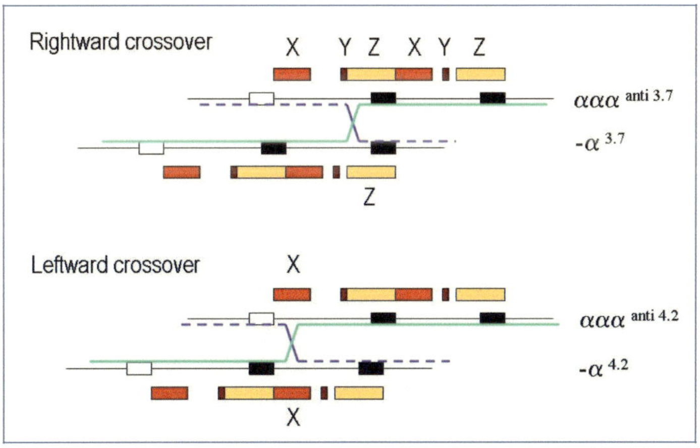

Figure 5. Schematic representation of α^+-thalassemia. $\alpha^{3.7}$ and $\alpha\alpha\alpha^{anti\ 3.7}$ chromosomes (top) resulting from rightward cross-over between the mis-paired Z boxes during meiosis. $-\alpha^{4.2}$ and $\alpha\alpha\alpha^{anti\ 4.2}$ chromosomes (bottom) resulting from leftward cross-over between misaligned X boxes [33]

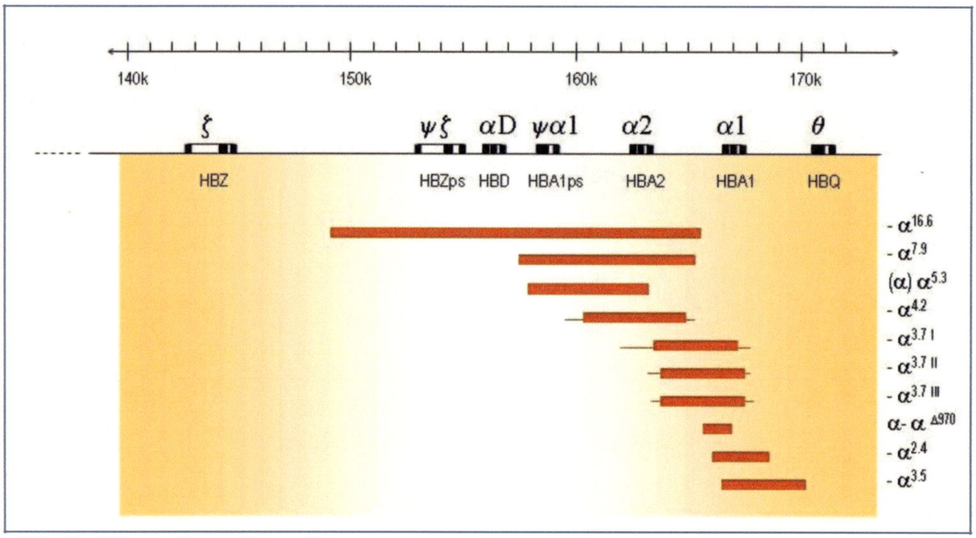

Figure 6. Deletions of one α-gene giving rise to α^{+}-thalassemia. The extent of the deletion is shown as bars, and thin lines indicate regions of uncertainty of the breakpoints [33]

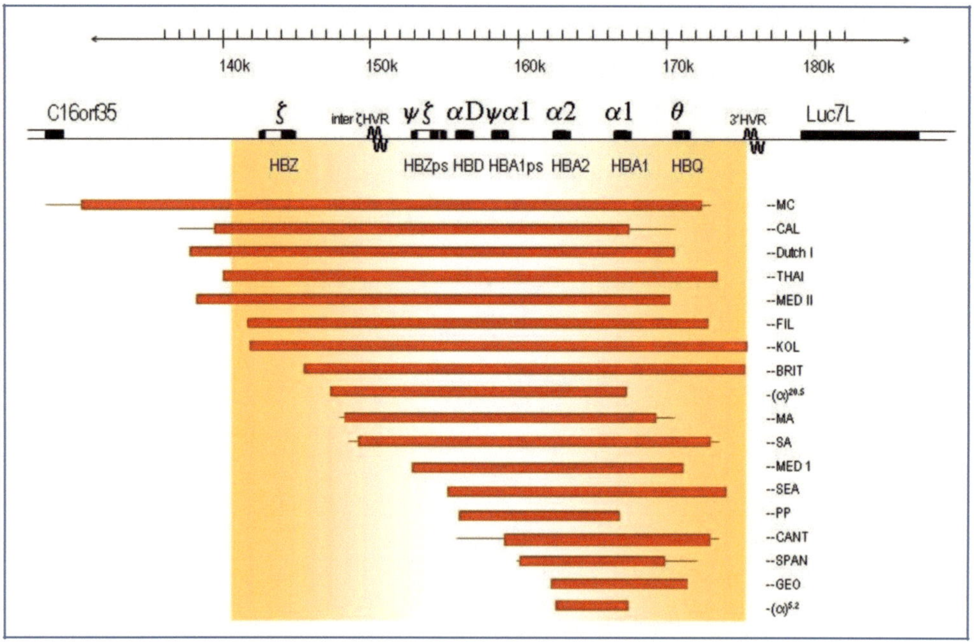

Figure 7. Deletions of two α-genes giving rise to α^{0}-thalassaemia [33]

- **α^{+}-thalassemia due to non-deletion types of α-thalassemia,** generally, the non-deletion α^{+}- thalassemia gives a more severe reduction in α-chain synthesis than the deletion type.

Many mutations have been described mostly affecting mRNA processing, translation, and α-globin stability. The most common non-deletional variants are the polyadenylation site mutations $\alpha^{2AATAAG}$, $\alpha^{2AATGAA}$, and $\alpha^{2AATA--}$ (Mediterranean and Middle East) [34,35].

- **α^0-thalassaemia due to deletions** many different length deletions have been found in patients with α^0 thalassemia, which were named after whom or where they were first discovered or by deletion size. The complete or partial deletion of both α-genes in *cis* results in no α-chain synthesis directed by these chromosomes *in vivo*. Homozygotes for such deletions have the Hb Bart's (Fig. 7&8) hydrops fetalis syndrome, while compound heterozygosity to the α° and α^+ defects results in a phenotype of hemoglobin H disease [19].

Some rare deletions of the regulatory region cause α^0-thalassaemia. This regulatory region lies 40–50 kb upstream of the α-globin gene cluster. This region composed of four multispecies conserved sequences (MCS), called MCS-R1 to R4, of which the most essential for α globin expression is MCS-R2 (HS-40) [36]. An overview showing all currently known $(\alpha\alpha)^T$ deletions is given in Figure 8 a and b.

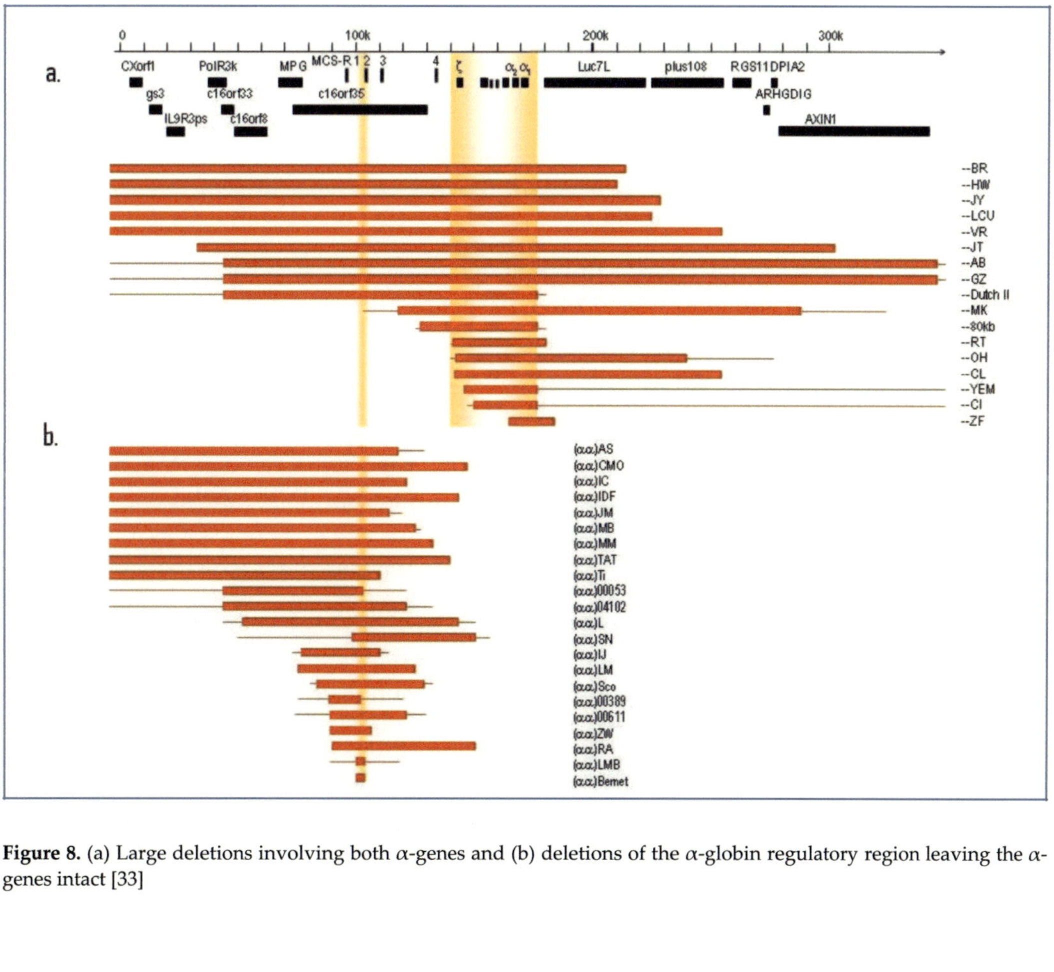

Figure 8. (a) Large deletions involving both α-genes and (b) deletions of the α-globin regulatory region leaving the α-genes intact [33]

α-thalassemia mental retardation X-linked (ATRX)

Hematologic malignancy and abnormal erythropoiesis may acquire changes in the hemoglobin structure or synthesis [Fig. 9]; however, the molecular basis of such abnormalities is obscure [5].

Somatic mutations in a known *trans*-acting regulator of globin gene expression were recently identified in patients with myelodysplasia, α-thalassemia mental retardation X-linked **(ATRX).** These new observations may increase the understanding of normal control of globin gene expression, as well as clarify common genetic or epigenetic mutations that contribute to the development or progression of myelodysplasia [5].

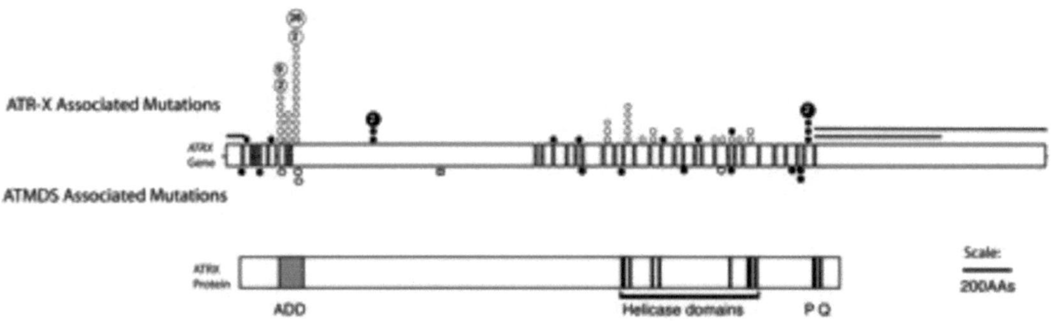

Figure 9. Schematic representation of the spectrum of *ATRX* mutations. Alignment of mutation sites in ATRX gene (top) with functionally important protein domains in ATRX protein (bottom) [5]

Genetic classification of β-thalassemia

The fact that only two genes encode the β-globin chain makes β-thalassemia simpler to understand than α-thalassemia. Unlike α-thalassemia, β-thalassemia rarely arises from the complete loss of a β-globin gene, but rather its suppression to variable degrees with essentially no beta globin protein production (β^0) or lower than normal (β^+). The severity of beta thalassemia depends in part on the type of β-thalassemic genes that a person has inherited.

- One β-globin gene affection; the residual production capacity of the defective beta globin gene tunes the degree of alpha-beta globin imbalance. One normally functioning beta gene, even if the other one produces no beta chain, would clinically present itself as mild anemia [37] that would be detected during a routine laboratory blood evaluation.

Two β-globin gene affection causes severe anemia and a potentially life-threatening condition. The severity of the disorder depends in part on the combination of genes that have been inherited: β^0thal/β^0thal; β^0thal/β^+thal; β^+thal/β^+thal, even though, the β^+ thalassemia genes vary greatly in their ability to produce normal hemoglobin.

β-thalassemias are heterogeneous at the molecular level. More than 300 disease-causing mutations have been identified so far. The distribution of β-thalassemia alleles varies highly from one population to another hence each population has its own spectrum of common B-thalassemia mutations that may be defined through a limited number of specific primers/

http://dx.doi.org/10.5772/61433

probes [38]. While most alleles behave as Mendelian recessives, there are variants that cause a disease phenotype even when present in a single copy.

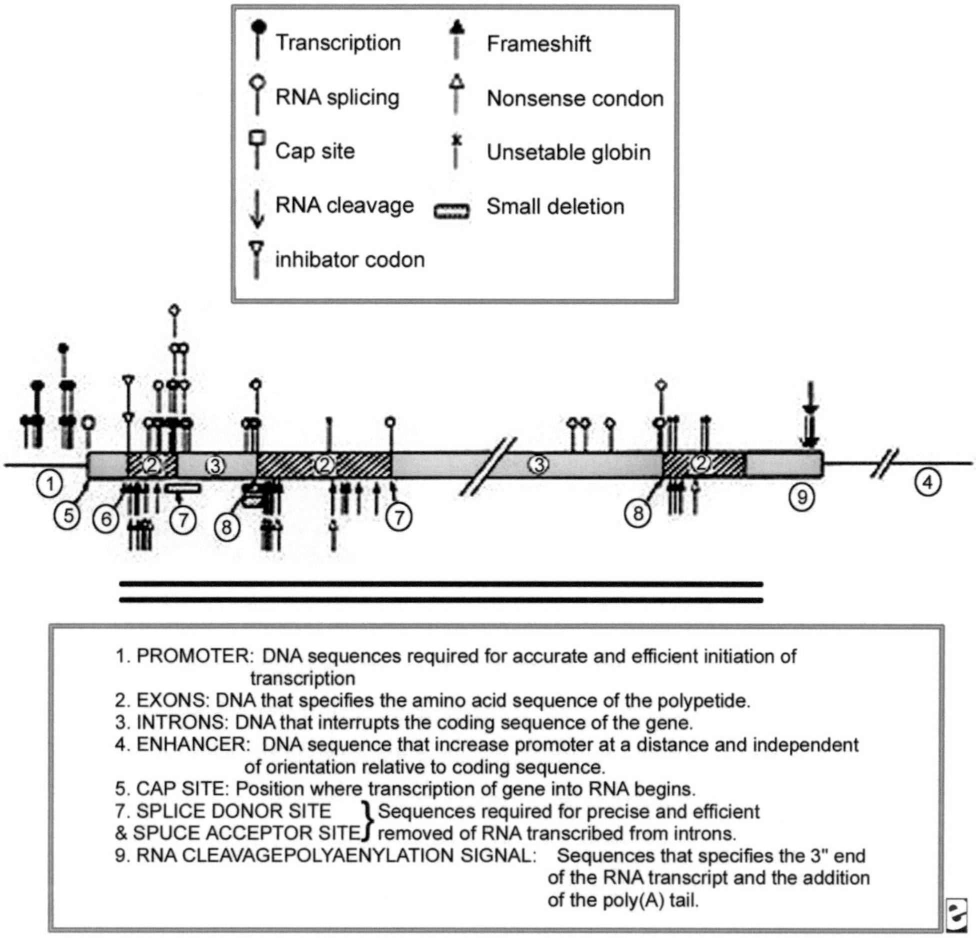

Figure 10. Beta globin gene mutations [39]

Most of reported beta globin gene mutations are single nucleotide substitutions or deletions or insertions (Fig.10) with consequent shift of reading frame. Gross gene deletion beta-thalassemias were reported in rare conditions. A complete updated list of beta-thalassemia mutations is available through the Globin Gene Server website [40]. β-thalassemia mutations may affect exonic intronic or the promoter (the 5′ and 3′ flanking UTR) sequences, accordingly affecting almost every known stage of the β-globin gene expression [23]. β-globin gene missense mutations, minor deletions leading to loss of intact codon, and frame shifts could all result in hyper unstable beta chains. Mutations producing the typical recessively inherited forms of β- thalassemia are located in exons 1 or 2 whereas most mutations in the phase termination codons that result in dominant beta-thalassemia lie in exon 3 [41].

In exons 1 or 2 mutations, a very small amount of beta globin mRNA is found in the cytoplasm of red blood cell precursors, whereas exon 3 mutations are associated with a substantial amount of abnormal cytoplasmic mRNA. This results in truncated unstable β- chain products, hence acting in a dominant-negative fashion, causing premature destruction of red blood cells. On the other hand, exons 1 and 2 premature termination codon mutations activate nonsense-mediated mRNA decay, thus precluding the accumulation of mRNA encoding for truncated peptides [41,42].

5. Different sorts of point mutations could affect β-globin expression

- **Transcriptional mutations**: described in each of the CACCC, CCAAT, and TATA boxes in the promoter region result in moderate reductions in transcription that give β^+ thalassemia with borderline reduced/normal red cell indices. Generally, such mutations are of β^+ or β^{++} mild forms of β-thalassemia.
- **RNA processing mutations**: the primary transcript of the β-globin gene is modified at the Cap site by the addition of a 7mG residue and at the 3′ end by an extension of 20–50 adenine residues, poly-A tail. A mutation of the cap site (+1 A → C) produces a mild form of β-thalassemia while numerous mutations of the poly-A addition signal result in more severe β^+ thalassemia in which normally modified mRNA is reduced to ~10% of normal [42].
- **Maturation of pre-mRNA:** if they fall into splicing or poly-adenylation sites. RNA splicing mutations represent a large portion of all β-thalassemia mutations; they affect the splicing process at variable degree, depending on mutation's position. Mutations occurring in the splicing consensus sequences are of β^+ type producing milder β-thalassemia. Whereas, mutations in exon or intron sequences may activate a cryptic splicing site leading to abnormal mRNA processing with defective splicing at variable degrees, and consequential mild to severe phenotypic affection [41,42].

Another group of splicing mutations involve nucleotide replacements within introns that create a new splice site that is used preferentially to the normal site. Depending on the strength of the new site these may result in either β^+ or β^0 thalassemia. Included in this group was the first characterized β-thalassemia allele, IVSI-110 G → A, the most common allele in the eastern Mediterranean region [42].

New splice sites may also be created by nucleotide substitutions in exons. These may also produce an amino acid change that would then produce an abnormal globin chain, leading to the production of reduced protein amounts.

- **Mutations affecting RNA stability**: occur in the 3′ or 5′ UTR, Cap site or the poly- adenylation site and are generally associated with mild β-thalassemia phenotypes. 5′ UTR mutations correlate with very mild phenotypes up to silent β-alleles with normal hematological phenotypes in heterozygotes [43].
- **Mutations affecting translation:** generate premature nonsense codons, premature termination of globin chain synthesis generally leads to the production of short, or to nonsense-

http://dx.doi.org/10.5772/61433

mediated decay (NMD) of abnormal mRNA. Six mutations of the translation initiation codon, AUG, have been described, all resulting in β^0 thalassemia. Downstream AUG sequences are not matched to the consensus sequence for translation initiation and would result in a shifted reading frame and a premature stop codon [44].

The deletion or insertion of one or a few nucleotides (other than multiples of three) into the coding region of the β globin gene causes a shift in the reading frame. These frame shift mutations will allow continued reading of an altered amino acid sequence until a new termination codon is reached, producing a truncated product that is non-functional [44].

6. Modifier genes and genotype-phenotype outcome

Phenotype-genotype studies aiming to unravel the clinical heterogeneity of beta thalassemia syndromes lead to the identification of a number of genetic factors that affect disease severity (Fig. 11 a&b).

a

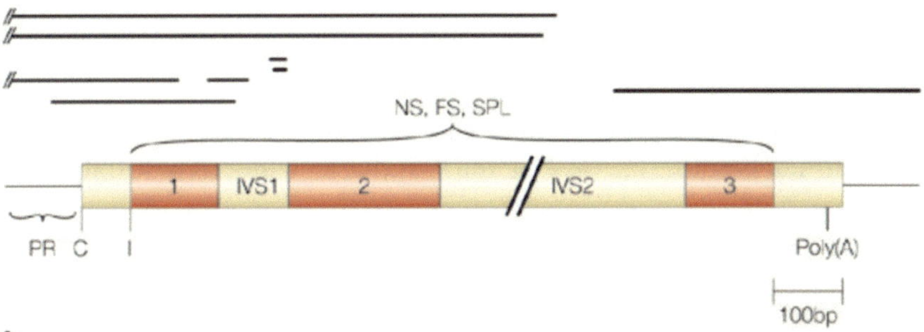

b

Mild β-thalassaemia alleles			'Silent' β-thalassaemia alleles
-90 C→T	-30 T→A	CD 26 G→A (Hb E)	-92 C→T
-88 C→A	-30 T→C	CD 27 G→T Knossos	-101 C→T
-88 C→T	-29 A→G	IVS1 6 T→C	5' UTR +10 -T
-87 C→A	-28 A→G (mild in blacks;	3' UTR 47 C→G	5' UTR +33 C→G
-87 C→G	severe in Chinese)	PolyA AATAAA→AACAAA	IVS2 844 C→G
-87 C→T	5' UTR +22 G→A	PolyA AATAAA→AATUAA	CAP +1 A→C
-86 C→G	CD 19 A→G Malay	PolyA AATAAA→AATAGA	3' UTR +6 C→G
-31 A→G	CD 24 T→A	PolyA AATAAA→AATAAC	

Figure 11. The effect of some beta globin mutations on phenotype.

Foremost among these is the nature of the β-globin mutations (primary modifiers) (Fig. 11). The major determinant of disease severity is the degree of β-globin chain deficit resulting from the nature of the β-thalassemia alleles.

As the phenotype correlates with α-globin chain deficiency and improved α/non-α chain imbalance, an increased residual level of HbF in adult life compensates the decreased β- globin chain, hence a major determinant of disease severity [45,46].

In the last few years, by application of genome wide association studies (GWAS), three major single nucleotide polymorphisms (SNPs) known as quantitative trait loci (QTL) that affect Hb F production levels were identified [47].

The first QTL is a SNP of unknown functional significance at position –158 (C>T) of the $^{G}\gamma$ promoter, called the XmnI polymorphism. The second locus is located on intron 2 of the BCL11A gene. The third locus is located between the HBS1L and MYB genes. It was suggested that the BCL11A and MYB proteins could act as γ-globin repressors [48].

Numerous polymorphisms located at the BCL11A gene on 2p16.18 and HBS1L-MYB intragenic region on 6q23.3 are either involved directly in fetal gene silencing in adult life or in cell proliferation and differentiation [49]. It was found that high-Hb F alleles at the BCL11A SNP (rs766432, rs4671393, rs1427407, and rs11886868) were significantly more frequent in patients with milder clinical forms of β-thalassemia and sickle cell disease (SCD), suggesting that this genetic polymorphism may be an important genetic modulator of disease severity [50]. Moreover, in the HBS1L-MYB intergenic region, different SNPs have been described as being associated with Hb F variations in different studies: rs9399137, rs4895441, rs9402686, and rs28384513 [51]. It was found that some particular tag-SNPs in these regions of favorable determinant are associated with high Hb F levels in healthy adults, as well as in thalassemia and SCD patients [52].

In $\delta\beta^0$ thalassemia, persistent production of gamma globin chains and their binding with α globin chains is an ameliorating factor. This ability is due to deletions of variable extents within the β-globin cluster, while in other cases it depends on the co-transmission of point mutations at $^{A}\gamma$ or $^{G}\gamma$ promoters (−196 C → T $^{A}\gamma$; −158 C → T XmnI SNP) [53,54].

Genetic modifiers are progressively used to explain different phenotypic expressions in two patients harboring the same beta-thalassemia mutation. These modifiers comprise factors affecting α- and β-chains imbalance in β-thalassemia, mainly the association of α-thalassemia deletions or mutations, with associated alleles contributing to the persistence and/or increased Hb F production after birth [55]. The evidence of mild phenotypes may also be determined by coinheritance of genetic determinants associated with increased γ- chain production mapping outside the β-globin cluster. It is expected that the identification of the role of genetic modifiers that modulate Hb F levels will shed light on the molecular mechanisms that control Hb F expression and on the etiology of the clinical heterogeneity observed in SCD patients [51,55].

Three different studies concerned with the association between the latter two QTLs with β-thalassemia concluded that predictions based on genetic modifiers could foresee the major or intermedia type of β-thalassemia, even in cohorts of patients with various β-globin genotypes, and that identification of the functional Hb F-QTL SNPs should help improve the accuracy of β-thalassemia major/β-thalassemia intermedia predictions [47,48,56].

Because of the major demographic changes in the pattern of disease in many of the developing countries, and the increased control of infant mortality due to diarrhea and infectious diseases, genetic diseases including thalassemias are floating on the surface as a health priority. Thus, translating the continuously growing molecular knowledge into readily understandable molecular pathology and extending molecular medicine is of utmost importance for disease control and management [9].

Although nearly all globin mutations characterized to date have been *cis*-acting defects, it has recently emerged that globin synthesis may also be altered by *trans*-acting mutations involving erythroid-specific and general transcriptional regulators [14,57].

Variable mutations of the globin genes has empowered researchers to use this system to launch many of the fundamental principles of human molecular genetics trying to improve our understanding of molecular hematology [14]. Hemoglobin synthesis is an excellent model for understanding mammalian gene regulation.

Studying the entire globin clusters through whole genome and/or exome analysis, among continuously emerging technical approaches of molecular biology, may be possible in the near future. New technologies may also allow rapid and far-reaching outlooks of partner genes playing a role in the regulation of hemoglobin synthesis.

Author details

Ghada Y. El-Kamah[1*] and Khalda S. Amr[2]

*Address all correspondence to: Ghadaelkamah@hotmail.com

1 Clinical Genetics department, Human Genetics & Genome Research Division, National Research Centre, Cairo, Egypt

2 Medical Molecular Genetics Department, Human Genetics & Genome Research Division, National Research Centre, Cairo, Egypt

References

[1] Salzano, F.M. & Maria, C.B. "Normal genetic variation at the protein, glycoconjugate and DNA levels", *The Evolution and Genetics of Latin American Populations*. 1st ed. Cambridge: Cambridge University Press, 2001. pp. 255-300. *Cambridge Books Online*. Web. 03 March 2015. http://dx.doi.org/10.1017/CBO9780511666100.009

[2] Weatherall, D.J. & Clegg, J.B. *The thalassaemia syndromes*. John Wiley & Sons, 2008.

[3] Weatherall, D.J. (2011). The inherited disorders of hemoglobin: an increasingly neglected global health burden. Indian J Med Res. 134(4), 493-497.

[4] http://www.news-medical.net/health/Thalassemia-Prevalence.aspx

[5] Steensma, D. P., Higgs, D. R., Fisher, C. A., & Gibbons, R. J. (2004). Acquired somatic ATRX mutations in myelodysplastic syndrome associated with α thalassemia

(ATMDS) convey a more severe hematologic phenotype than germline ATRX mutations. *Blood, 103*(6), 2019-2026.

[6] Caro A , Galanello R , Origa R(2000). Beta-Thalassemia, Gene Reviews Initial Posting: September 28; Last Update: January 24, 2013.

[7] http://web2.airmail.net/uthman/hemoglobinopathy/globin_chromosomes.gif

[8] Schechter, A.N., (2008). Hemoglobin research and the origins of molecular medicine. Blood; 112: 3927-3938.

[9] Weatherall D.J. & Clegg J.B. The Thalassaemia syndromes. 4th ed. Oxford, U.K: Blackwell Science Ltd; 2001. CrossRef. Weatherall DJ, Clegg JB and Naughton MA (1965) Globin synthesis in thalassemia: an in vitro study. Nature 208: 1061-1065.

[10] Weatherall DJ, Clegg JB, Higgs DR, Wood WG (1989). The Hemoglobinopathies. USA: McGraw-Hill.

[11] Amoako, Y. A., & Bedu-Addo, G. (2014). Hyper-reactive Malarial Splenomegaly (HMS) in a patient with ² thalassaemia syndrome. *Pan African Medical Journal, 19* (310), 19-25.

[12] Shinar, E., & Rachmilewitz, E. A. (1990). Oxidative denaturation of red blood cells in thalassemia. In *Seminars in hematology*. 27(1), 70-82.

[13] Nathan, D. G., & Gunn, R. B. (1966). Thalassemia: the consequences of unbalanced hemoglobin synthesis. *The American journal of medicine, 41*(5), 815-830.

[14] Steensma, D. P., Gibbons, R. J., & Higgs, D. R. (2005). Acquired α-thalassemia in association with myelodysplastic syndrome and other hematologic malignancies. *Blood, 105*(2), 443-452.

[15] Waye, J. S., & Chui, D. H. (2001). The alpha-globin gene cluster: genetics and disorders. *Clinical and investigative medicine, 24*(2), 103-109.

[16] Padraic P. Levings, Bungert J.(2002). The Human Globin Locus Control Region. A Center Of Attraction. Eur. J. Biochem. 269, 1589-1599.

[17] Chui D.H. (2005). Alpha-thalassemia: Hb H disease and Hb Barts hydrops fetalis. *Ann N Y Acad Sci.* 1054, 25-32.

[18] Piel, F. B., & Weatherall, D. J. (2014). The α-Thalassemias. *N Engl J Med, 371,* 1908-16.

[19] Al-Allawi, N. A., Shamdeen, M. Y., Rasheed, N. S. (2010). Homozygosity for the Mediterranean α-thalassemic deletion (hemoglobin Barts hydrops fetalis). *Annals of Saudi Medicine. 30*(2), 153.

[20] Vichinsky, E.P. (2005). Changing Patterns of Thalassemia Worldwide. *Ann N Y Acad Sci.* 1054, 18–24.

[21] Danjou, F., Anni, F., Galanello, R. (2011). Beta-thalassemia: from genotype to phenotype. *Haematologica, 96*(11), 1573-1575.

[22] Bouva, M. J., Harteveld, C. L., van Delft, P., Giordano, P. C. (2006). Known and new delta globin gene mutations and their diagnostic significance. *Haematologica. 91*(1), 129-132.

[23] http://www.ncbi.nlm.nih.gov/omim. (MIM# 142000, 141749, 141900)

[24] Forget, B. G. (1998). Molecular basis of hereditary persistence of fetal hemoglobin. *Annals of the New York Academy of Sciences, 850*(1), 38-44.

[25] Sukumaran, P. K., Nakatsuji, T., Gardiner, M. B., Reese, A. L., Gilman, J. G., Huisman, T. H. (1983). Gamma thalassemia resulting from the deletion of a gamma-globin gene. *Nucleic Acids Research. 11*(13), 4635–4643.

[26] Olivieri, N. F., Pakbaz, Z., Vichinsky, E. (2011). Hb E/beta-thalassaemia: a common & clinically diverse disorder. *The Indian Journal of Medical Research. 134*(4), 522–531.

[27] Mukherjee, M. B., Nadkarni, A. H., Gorakshakar, A. C., Ghosh, K., Mohanty, D., Colah, R. B. (2010). Clinical, hematologic and molecular variability of sickle cell-β thalassemia in western India. *Indian Journal of Human Genetics. 16*(3), 154–158.

[28] Saleh-gohari, N. & Mohammadi-Anaie, M. (2012). Co-Inheritance of Sickle Cell Trait and Thalassemia Mutations in South Central Iran. *Iranian Journal of Public Health. 41*(10), 81–86.

[29] Piel, F. B., Howes, R. E., Patil, A. P., Nyangiri, O. A., Gething, P. W., Bhatt, S., ... Hay, S. I. (2013). The distribution of haemoglobin C and its prevalence in newborns in Africa. *Scientific Reports. 3*, 1671.

[30] Zakarenia M, Ayatollahi M, Rastegar M, Amanat Sh, Askarinejad AR, Amirghofran S, Hagheshenas M. (2011). Hemoglobin D (HbD Punjab/ Los Angeles and HbD Iran) and co-inheritance of Alpha- and Beta- Thalassemia in Southern Iran. Iranian Red Crescent Medical Journal. 13(7), 493-498.

[31] Chehab, F., (2010). Molecular Diagnostic Challenges of the Thalassemias. chapter 36.Molecular Diagnostics: Techniques and Applications for the Clinical Laboratory 1 ed. By Academic Press. Inc. 441-452.

[32] Trent, R.J., Higgs, D.R., Clegg, J.B., Weatherall, D.J. (1981). A new triplicated a-globin gene arrangement in man. Br. J. haematol. 49, 149.

[33] Harteveld, C.L. and Higgs, D.R. (2010): α-thalassemia. *Orphanet Journal of Rare Diseases*. 5, 13.

[34] Harteveld CL, Losekoot M, Haak H, Heister GA, Giordano PC, Bernini LF (1994): A novel polyadenylation signal mutation in the alpha 2-globin gene causing alpha thalassaemia. *Br J Haematol*, 87:139-143.

[35] Higgs DR, Goodbourn SE, Lamb J, Clegg JB, Weatherall DJ, Proudfoot NJ (1983): Alpha-thalassaemia caused by a polyadenylation signal mutation. *Nature*, 306:398-400.

[36] Higgs DR (2009): The molecular basis of alpha -thalassemia. In Disorders of Hemoglobin second edition. Edited by: Steinberg MH, Forget BG, Higgs DR, Nagel RL. *Cambridge University Press.*

[37] Sharma S, Raina V, Chandra J, Narayan S, Sharma S. (2006). Lupus anticoagulant and anticardiolipin antibodies in polytransfused beta thalassemia major. Hematology. 11(4): 287-290.

[38] Finotti, A. & Gambari, R. (2014). Recent trends for novel options in experimental biological therapy of β-thalassemia. *Expert Opinion on Biological Therapy.14*(10), 1443-1454.

[39] http://img.medscape.com/pi/emed/ckb/pediatrics_general/1331341-1331366-958850-959073.jpg, (2013).

[40] http://www.globin.cse.psu.edu (2015).

[41] Cao A. and Galanello R. (2010). Beta-thalassemia. *Genetics in Medicine* .12 (2); 61–76.

[42] Wood, B. & Higgs, D.R. (2009). Molecular basis of thalassemia syndromes. ESH Handbook on Disorders of Erythropoiesis, Erythrocytes and Iron Metabolism. 250–263.

[43] Khan J. (2014) Molecular Basis of Thalassemia Intermedia in Pakistan. JSM Cell Dev Biol. 2(2): 1010

[44] Peixeiro, I., Silva, A.L., Romão, L. (2011). Control of human β-globin mRNA stability and its impact on beta-thalassemia phenotype. *Haematologica. 96*(6), 905–913.

[45] El-Kamah, G. Y., Hosny, L. A., Sobh, H. A. (2009). Exploring Phenotypic Alterations in Response to High Hemoglobin F Level in Egyptian Beta Thalassemia Patients. *Journal of Applied Sciences Research, 5*(10).

[46] Thein, S.L., Menzel, S., Lathorp, M., Garner, C. (2009). Control of fetal hemoglobin: new insights emerging from genomics and clinical implications. Hum Mol Genet. 18(R2), 216-223.

[47] Banan, M. (2013). Hydroxyurea treatment in β-thalassemia patients: to respond or not to respond? Ann Hematol. 92(3), 289–299.

[48] Badens, C., Joly, P., Agouti, I., Thuret I., Gonnet, K., Fattoum S., Francina, A., Simeoni, M., Loundou, A., Pissard, S. (2011). Variants in genetic modifiers of β-thalassemia can help to predict the major or intermedia type of the disease. Haematologica. 96(11), 1712–1714.

[49] Galarneau, G., Palmer, C.D., Sankaran, V.S., Orkin, S.H., Hirschhorn, J.N., Lettre, G. (2010). Fine-mapping at three loci known to affect fetal hemoglobin levels explains additional genetic variation. Nat Genet. 42(12), 1049–1051.

[50] Uda, M., Galanello, R., Sanna, S., Lettre, G., Sankaran, V.G., Chen, W., Usala, G., Busonero, F., Maschio, A., Albai, G., Piras, M.G., Sestu, N., Lai, S., Dei, M., Mulas, A., Crisponi, L., Naitza, S., Asunis, I., Deiana, M., Nagaraja, R., Perseu, L., Satta, S., Cipollina, M.D., Sollaino, C., Moi, P., Hirschhorn, J.N., Orkin, S.H., Abecasis, G.R., Schlessinger, D., Cao A. (2008). Genome-wide association study shows BCL11A associated with persistent fetal hemoglobin and amelioration of the phenotype of beta-thalassemia. Proc Natl Acad Sci U S A. 105(5),1620-5.

[51] Lettre, G.; Sankaran, V.G., BEZERRA, m.A.c., Araûjo, A.S., Uda, M., Sanna, S, Cao, A., Schlessinger, D., Costa, F.F., Hirschhorn, J.N., ORKIN, S.H. (2008). DNA polymorphisms at the BCL11A, HBS1L-MYB, and β-globin loci associate with fetal hemoglobin levels and pain crises in sickle cell disease. Proc Natl Acad Sci U S A, 105(33), 11869-11874.

[52] So, C.C., Song, Y.Q., et al. (2008). The HBS1L-MYB intergenic region on chromosome 6q23 is a quantitative trait locus controlling fetal haemoglobin level in carriers of β-thalassaemia. J Med Genet, 45, No. 11, (Nov), pp 745-775.

[53] Tasiopoulou, M., Boussiou, M., Sinopoulou, K., Moraitis, G., Loutradi-Anagnostou, A., Karababa, P.G. (2008). Gamma-196 C-->T, A gamma-201 C-->T: two novel mutations in the promoter region of the gamma-globin genes associated with nondeletional hereditary persistence of fetal hemoglobin in Greece. Blood Cells Mol Dis. 40(3), 320–322.

[54] Labie, D., Dunda-Belkhodja, O., Rouabhi, F., Pagnier, J., Ragusa, A., Nagel, R.L. (1985). The -158 site 5′ to the G gamma gene and G gamma expression. Blood. 66(6), 1463–1465.

[55] El-Kamah, G. Y., El-Beshlawy, A., Sobh, H. A., & Hussein, I. R. (2003). Phenotypic scoring in thalassemia intermedia and the impact of underlying molecular defects. *Med J Cairo Univ*, 4(Suppl II), 323-327.

[56] Galanello, R., Sanna S., Perseu, L., Sollaino, M.C., Satta, S., Lai, M.E., Barella, S., Uda, M, Usala, G., Abecasis, G.R., Cao, A. (2009). Amelioration of Sardinian β0 thalassemia by genetic modifiers. Blood. 114(18), 3935-3937.

[57] Nichols, K. E., Crispino, J. D., Poncz, M., White, J. G., Orkin, S. H., Maris, J. M., & Weiss, M. J. (2000). Familial dyserythropoietic anaemia and thrombocytopenia due to an inherited mutation in GATA1. *Nature genetics*, *24*(3), 266-270.

Chapter 3

Sickle Cell Disease (SCD)

Ahmed K. Mansour, Sohier Yahia, Rasha El-Ashry, Angi Alwakeel,
Ahmad Darwish and Khalil Alrjjal

Additional information is available at the end of the chapter

http://dx.doi.org/10.5772/61162

Abstract

Sickle cell anemia (SCA) is a disease that is caused by the formation of an abnormal hemoglobin type, which can bind with other abnormal hemoglobin molecules within the red blood cells (RBCs) to cause rigid distortion of the cell. This distortion prevents the cell from passing through small blood vessels; leading to occlusion of vascular beds, followed by tissue ischemia and infarction. Infarction is frequent all over the body in patients with SCA, leading to the acute pain crisis. Over time, such insults result in medullary bone infarcts and epiphyseal osteonecrosis. In the brain, cognitive impairment and functional neurologic deficits may occur due to white matter and gray matter infarcts. Infarction may also affect the lungs increasing susceptibility to pneumonia. The liver, spleen, and kidney may show infarction as well. Sequestration crisis is an unusual life-threatening complication of SCA, in which a significant amount of blood is sequestered in an organ (usually the spleen), leading to collapse. Lastly, since the RBCs are abnormal, they are destroyed, resulting in a hemolytic anemia. However, the ischemic complications in patients with SCA disease far exceed the anemia in clinical significance.

Keywords: Sickle, update, hydroxyuria

1. Introduction

1.1. Hemoglobinopathies

Hemoglobin is needed for transfer of oxygen to different body organs. The shape of the red blood cell can be affected by the type of the hemoglobin. Hemoglobinopathies are hemoglobin abnormalities that influence its formation. The severity of these disorders varies widely and can lead to death. Hemolytic anemia is a common presentation for hemoglobinopathies. Sickle cell anemia is one of these hemoglobinopathies.

1.2. Definition of sickle cell anemia

Sickle cell anemia is an inherited disease characterized by the presence of an abnormal hemoglobin called hemoglobin S (HbS). During deoxygenation, the red blood cell (RBC) shape changes from the biconcave shape to the sickle shape due to the abnormal hemoglobin. The shape of the RBC changes back to the biconcave shape after reoxygenation. However, the frequent sickling and unsickling leads to hemolysis and anemia. [1]

1.3. Inheritance of hemoglobinopathies

There are three types of normal hemoglobin: hemoglobin A (HbA), hemoglobin F (HbF), and hemoglobin A_2 (HbA_2). Each hemoglobin molecule contains four polypeptide chains that differ from one type to another. Hemoglobin A contains 2 alpha globin chains and two beta globin chains and comprises 95–97% of the normal hemoglobin. Hemoglobin A_2 contains 2 alpha globin chains and two gamma globin chains and comprises 2.5–3.5% of the normal hemoglobin. Hemoglobin F contains 2 alpha globin chains and two delta globin chains and comprises <1% of the normal hemoglobin. The gene coding for the α globin chain is sited on chromosome 16, however, the non-α globin gene cluster is located on chromosome 11. [2,3]

There is a transversion mutation at the sixth codon of the β globin gene from A to T which produces HbS, with a substitution at the 6th amino acid position in the β globin polypeptide chain to be valine instead of glutamic acid. Patients with sickle cell anemia (homozygous to HbS gene) have HbS instead of HbA associated with formation of HbF and HbA_2. Some patients with sickle cell disease (double heterozygous) have got HbS together with other types of abnormal hemoglobin or even they are sickle-thalassemia. However, thalassemias on their own occur more frequently giving rise to homozygous disease conditions.[4]Abnormal hemoglobin is responsible for hemolysis and vaso-occlusion that can lead to tissue infarction. [5,6]

1.4. Pattern of inheritance of hemoglobinopathies

Hemoglobin abnormalities and the thalassemias are inherited as autosomal recessive (AR) disorders, where carrier parents transmit the disease to their offspring. If both parents are heterozygotes for HbS, there is a 25 per cent chance of having a homozygous HbSS (Sickle cell anemia, SCA) child. A double heterozygote state occurs when one parent is a heterozygote for HbS and the other is heterozygote for one of the abnormal HbS or thalassemias. Heterozygotes are asymptomatic carriers (traits), while the SCD is presented in the homozygotes and the double heterozygotes for two abnormal hemoglobin genes or HbS and the thalassemias.[6]

1.5. Pathophysiology of sickle cell anemia

Sickle cell anemia is a single gene disorder which is produced by a point mutation in the beta globin gene which is found on chromosome 11. This leads to replacement of glutamic acid (a hydrophilic amino acid) in the sixth position with valine (a hydrophobic amino acid). [7] Hemoglobin S is formed from the association of two α-globin subunits with two mutant β-globin subunits. On exposure to hypoxic conditions, the absence of a polar amino acid at position six of the β-globin chain encourages the non-covalent polymerization (aggregation)

http://dx.doi.org/10.5772/61162

of hemoglobin, which changes the shape and elasticity of RBCs.In low oxygen media, the cells attain an abnormal shape which is not elastic. When normal oxygen tension is regained, the cells fail to return to their normal shape. Therefore, these distorted RBCs cannot pass through narrow capillaries, leading to occlusion of blood vessels. Vaso-occlusion results in hand-foot syndrome in children. Furthermore, infections, stroke, and acute chest pain are some of the major complications. Most of these complications start in early life, but become clearer with advancing age. Infections, dehydration, cold weather, and stress are considered as precipitating factors for these complications. Treatments of SCD are mostly directed toward prevention of or decreasing sickling and thus reducing the incidence of vascular occlusion. [5-10]

The abnormal shape of the RBCs leads to their destruction by hemolysis. A compensatory bone marrow hyperplasia is not able to match the rate of RBC destruction.[8] Sickle cells only survive 10–20 days in comparison to normal RBCs which typically live 90–120 days.[9]

2. Epidemiology of sickle cell gene

Sickle cell anemia is most common among people from Africa, India, the Caribbean, the Middle East, and the Mediterranean. In the Middle East, the first report of HbS and thalassemias came from Egypt. [11,12] The presence of HbS in Eastern Saudi Arabia was reported by Lehmann. [13] Many studies on hemoglobinopathies have been documented from most countries of the Middle East. Table (1) presents a brief history for identification of abnormal hemoglobins in the Middle East. HbS is the major variant identified in all areas. [14]

Discovery country	Year
First case of SCD in Egypt	1951
HbS in Middle East	1959
HbO-Arab in Egyptian family	1960
HbS in Saudi Arabia	1963
HbS and HbO-Arab in Sudan	1966
HbC in Egyptians	1967
Mild SCD in Saudi Arabia	1969
SCD in Kuwait	1969
HbH disease in Kuwait	1969
HbS in Egyptian western desert	1974
HbC in Libya	1975
HbS in Abu Dhabi	1980
HbC in Saudi Arabia	1979
HbE and HbD in Abu Dhabi	1979
HbO-Arab in Saudi Arabia	1980
HbS. α- and β-thal in several regions of Saudi Arabia	1967–1982

Table 1. Hemoglobinopathies in the Middle East Arab countries

3. Clinical manifestations of sickle cell anemia

Sickle cell anemia presents with severe hemolytic anemia interrupted by crises. Symptoms of anemia in SCD are often mild in relation to the severity of the anemia because HbS gives up oxygen (O_2) to tissues relatively easily compared with HbA, its O_2 dissociation curve is shifted to the right (see Figure 1). [15]

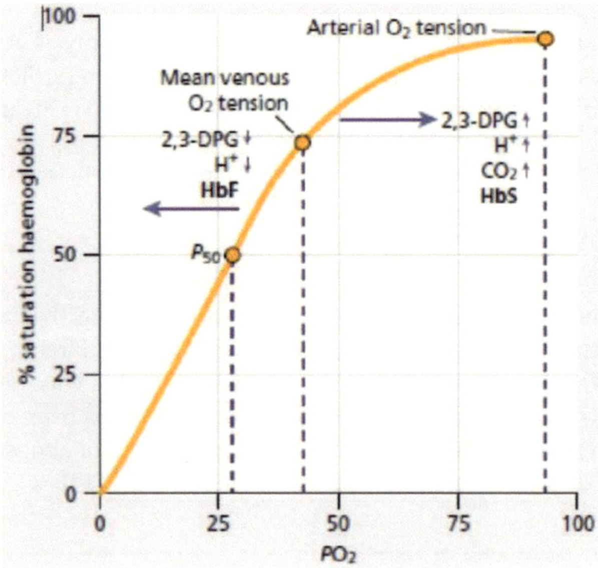

Figure 1. The hemoglobin oxygen dissociation curve. 2,3-DPG, 2,3-diphosphoglycerate.

The clinical presentation of SCD is variable, with some patients having a normal life; however, some patients show increased morbidity and mortality due to severe thrombotic, aplastic, and sequestration crises. [15]

3.1. Vaso-occlusive crises

The vaso-occlusive crises are the commonest. Their etiology is usually attributed to low oxygen tension as in high altitude, water loss, and infection. Vaso-occlusion leads to severe pain especially in bones (hips, shoulders, and vertebrae) (Figures 2–4). [15] Infarcts of the small bones lead to painful dactylitis (hand-foot syndrome). It is usually the first presentation of the disease and may lead to digits of varying lengths (Figure 4). [15] Soft tissues affected include the lungs and the spleen. The most serious vaso-occlusive crisis is of the brain (a stroke occurs in 7% of all patients) or spinal cord.

Transcranial Doppler ultrasonography detects abnormal blood flow indicative of arterial stenosis. This can predict the occurrence of strokes in children.[15]

http://dx.doi.org/10.5772/61162

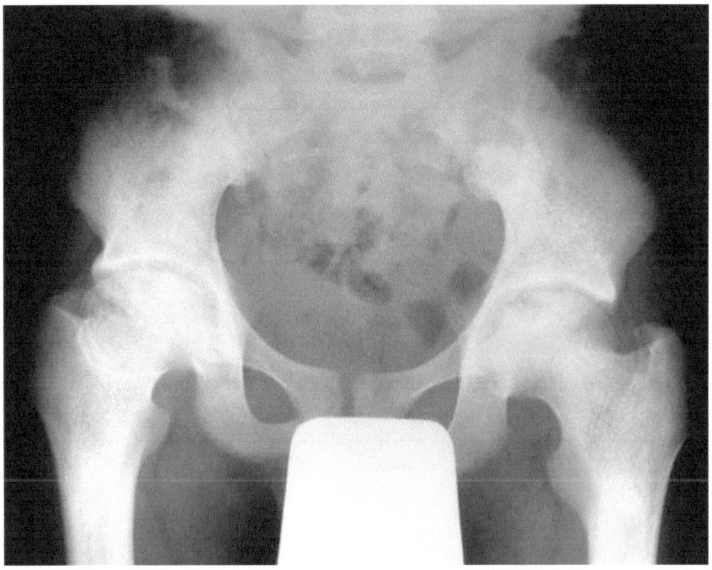

Figure 2. Radiograph of the pelvis of a young man of West Indian origin, which shows avascular necrosis with flattening of the femoral heads, more marked on the right hip, coarsening of the bone architecture, and cystic areas in the right femoral neck caused by previous infarcts.

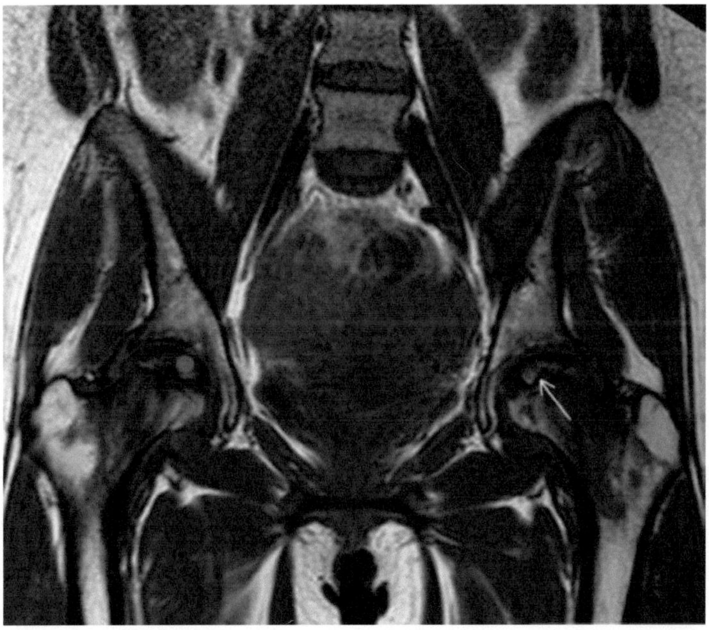

Figure 3. Sickle cell anemia. Coronal hip MRI image revealing established osteonecrosis of femoral heads bilaterally (yellow arrow) with crescentric sclerotic margin (blue dot) as a consequence of sickle cell disease (Courtesy of Dr A. Malhotra).

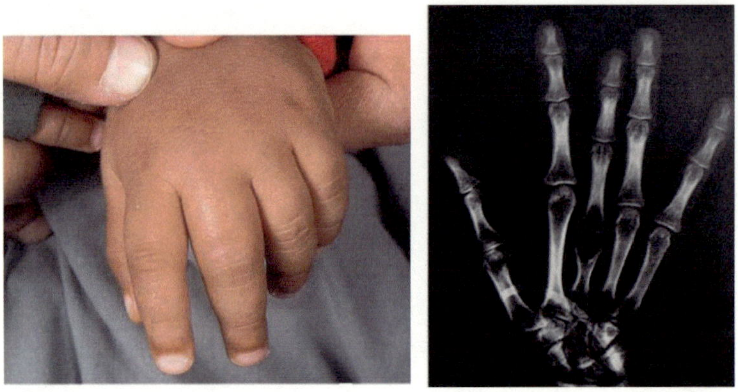

Figure 4. Sickle cell anemia: **(a)** painful swollen fingers (dactylitis) in a child; and **(b)** the hand of an 18-year-old Nigerian boy with the ' hand - foot ' syndrome. There is marked shortening of the right middle finger because of dactylitis in childhood affecting the growth of the epiphysis..

3.2. Sequestration crises

These crises are caused by pooling of blood, with severe exacerbation of anemia. The acute sickle chest syndrome is the most common cause of death after puberty. The patients present with dyspnea, arterial hypoxia, chest pain, and lung infiltrates on chest X-ray. Treatment includes analgesics, oxygen, exchange transfusion, and ventilator support if needed. Hepatic and splenic sequestration may lead to severe disease necessitating exchange transfusion. The splenic sequestration is characteristically found in infants and clinically presents with an enlarging spleen, decreased hemoglobin, and abdominal pain. The patients are treated mainly with blood transfusion, and they must be monitored frequently as rapid progression may occur. The crises are usually recurrent and the patient is usually in need of splenectomy. [15]

3.2.1. Aplastic crises

Aplastic crises are due to parvovirus infection and are characterized by a sudden fall in hemoglobin, usually requiring transfusion. The patient shows anemia together with reticulocytopenia. [15]

3.2.2. Hemolytic crises

In these crises, the patients show a higher rate of hemolysis with a decline in hemoglobin level associated with reticulocytosis. Hemolytic crises usually accompany vaso-occlusive crises.

3.2.3. Other clinical features

Chronic hemolytic anemia is the main clinical presentation of SCD with recurrent attacks of acute painful vaso-occlusive crises. SCD is also associated with multi-organ acute and chronic complications. The clinical features of SCD are summarized in Table (2). The size of the spleen is increased during infancy and early childhood but later is usually decreased due to infarction (autosplenectomy). Pulmonary hypertension and tricuspid regurgitation may occur and increases the risk of mortality. Retinopathy and priapism may also complicate the course of patients with SCD. Chronic liver damage may occur due to microinfarction associated with gall bladder stones. Renal medullary infarction with papillary necrosis may be present in the course of sickle cell anemia. The ability of the kidney to concentrate urine may be lost leading to dehydration and vaso- occlusive crises, and nocturnal enuresis is common. [15]

Although the genetic aberration in SCD is precisely well understood, there is a clear variability in the clinical severity of the disease among patients. Some patients lead a normal life, free of problems; others may show severe crises or have fatal complications. The life expectancy of patients with SCD is decreased but is increasing due to the improvement in supportive therapies, especially prophylactic antibiotics, stroke screening in early childhood, increased administration of hydroxycarbamide or transfusion, and improved care. Intensive care is needed for patients complicated by acute chest syndrome (ACS), acute stroke, or acute renal injury.[16]

Complication	Clinical presentation
Painful crisis	These crises occur in most of patients with SCD; they are variable in frequency and severity May lead to a chronic pain syndrome
Neurological	Microvascular occlusion may be seen on MRI. May lead to cognitive disability. Stroke affects 10% of children; it is a leading cause of morbidity and mortality. Can be prevented by regular blood transfusion
Pulmonary	Acute chest syndrome Asthma, fibrotic lung disease The main cause of death in adults, high risk of acute respiratory failure There is an increased association with airway hyperactivity.
Gastrointestinal Cholelithiasis Hepatopathy	Most patients have gall bladder stones due to hemolysis Decompensated liver disease may be present in some patients
Renal, Urological	Chronic renal failure occurs in 20% of patients Priapism may be present leading to sexual dysfunction
Ophthalmology	Proliferative retinopathy is common in patients with HbSC disease
Orthopedic Avascular necrosis Osteomyelitis	Common complication of hip and shoulders, requiring replacement Salmonella is the most common organism
Hematological Hemolytic anemia Aplastic crisis Splenic sequestration	Chronic hemolysis, usual Hb 6–9 g/dL, higher in HbSC Parvovirus B19 infection may trigger red cell aplasia. The combination of red cell aplasia and hemolysis can be fatal Typically seen in infants with a rapidly enlarging spleen

Table 2. Clinical presentation of sickle cell disease (SCD)

3.3. Diagnosis

In HbSS, the complete blood count shows hemoglobin levels in the range of 6-8 g/dL with reticulocytosis (due to compensatory bone marrow hyperplasia). In other forms of sickle-cell disease, Hb levels tend to be higher. A blood film may reveal sickle shaped cells and features of hyposplenism (target cells and Howell-Jolly bodies) (Figure 5). [15]

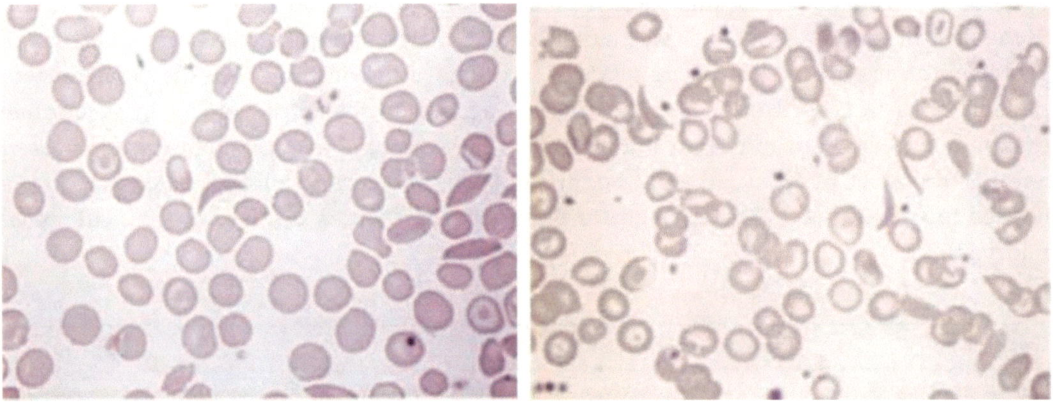

Figure 5. Sickle cell anemia: peripheral blood films showing deeply staining sickle cells, target cells and polychromasia.

Hemoglobin electrophoresis is used to diagnose the presence of abnormal hemoglobin types. Hemoglobin S and hemoglobin SC are the two most common forms detected in sickle cell-diseased patients. High-performance liquid chromatography (HPLC) is used to confirm the diagnosis. Genetic study is not frequently done as electrophoresis and HPLC are accurate in detecting HbS and HbC.[17]

Infection may precipitate the acute sickle-cell crisis. Therefore, a urinalysis to detect an occult urinary tract infection, and chest X-ray to look for occult pneumonia should be performed.[18]

Genetic counseling is usually needed for carriers of SCD before they have a child. Fetal blood sampling or amniocentesis can be done to see if the fetus has the disease. Miscarriage is more common with fetal blood sampling than with amniocentesis.

4. General principles of management of SCD

Crises management is usually supportive unless blood transfusion is indicated. The aim of treatment is to prevent the sickling of RBCs, dehydration, hypoxia, and acidosis that can induce sickling. Painful attack is the main presentation. Subcutaneous morphine or another strong opiate is frequently required for management of severe attacks of pain. Pethidine can precipitate Grand mal seizures; therefore, it is preferable to be avoided. Satisfactory fluid intake is mandatory.

4.1. Folic acid and penicillin

Children born with sickle-cell disease will take folic acid (1 mg dose) daily for life. In addition, Patients from birth to five years of age have to take penicillin daily due to susceptibility to pneumococcal infection.

4.2. Acute chest syndrome

Acute chest syndrome is an acute illness with fever and/or respiratory symptoms associated with a new lung infiltrate. It is the main cause of mortality in adults with SCD and the most common cause of intensive care unit admission. The patient who needs mechanical ventilation is reported to have a mortality rate of 5%.[16] Symptoms include cough, wheeze, dyspnea, and chest pain, which may be pleuritic or affect the ribs and sternum. The acute chest syndrome is unique to SCD and is associated with a more severe course and worse outcome than pneumonia.

Blood transfusion is used to treat patients with acute chest syndrome and will improve the oxygenation. Blood transfusion is useful in less severe cases with a low Hb (<7 g/dL); however, exchange transfusion is needed in severe cases, in patients with high Hb levels, or those with severe hypoxia. The target is a final Hb level of 9–10 g/dL. Severe hypoxia, dyspnea and respiratory acidosis are indications for initiating advanced respiratory support.[19]

4.3. Stroke

Patients with SCD are commonly associated with ischemic and hemorrhagic strokes, with a prevalence rate of more than 5%. Incidence of stroke is greatly reduced after the introduction of transcranial Doppler screening and primary stroke prevention with transfusion. A stroke may be precipitated by dehydration or a coincident illness.

Early imaging is essential to confirm the diagnosis and exclude hemorrhage. MRI is the imaging of choice with high sensitivity and specificity. If the MRI confirms a stroke, immediate exchange transfusion should be done to achieve an HbS less than 30%. Ischemic stroke prevention can be done by long-term exchange transfusion, however the efficacy of antiplatelet therapy in primary or secondary stroke prevention in SCD is not proved.[20]

4.4. Sepsis

Patients with sickle cell anemia have functional hyposplenism. This makes them more susceptible to infection by capsulated organisms. Sepsis caused by gram-negative organisms is common together with osteomyelitis. Children with sickle cell anemia have to be vaccinated against pneumococcal, meningococcal, and *Hemophilus influenza* infection. Oral penicillin could be given on daily basis after the time of diagnosis to guard against pneumococcal infection. [21]

4.5. Other complications of SCD

Patients with SCD have low renal concentrating ability and are therefore susceptible to dehydration. Over time, the patients may show proteinuria and chronic renal impairment as a result of glomerular damage. This leaves patients liable to acute kidney injury during a crisis. Chronic lung disease is common and manifests as either a restrictive lung defect or an overnight hypoxia and sleep apnea. Pulmonary hypertension is more common in SCD and can lead to marked hypoxia.[16]

4.5.1. Admission to critical care unit

Patients with sickle cell anemia may need admission to the intensive care unit either due to liver cell failure, sepsis, or multi-organ damage. This acute deterioration may necessitate urgent blood transfusion aiming for an Hb of 9–10 g/dL and HbS% of less than 30%. This will improve tissue oxygenation and perfusion, whatever the underlying etiology.[22]

4.5.2. Transfusion in SCD patients

Regular blood transfusion is needed to prevent brain strokes. Special situations such as circulatory disturbances, sequestration crises and priapism may need blood transfusion to optimize oxygen transport. [23]

Partial exchange transfusion is usually preferred to simple transfusion if routine or multiple transfusions are necessary. It decreases the iron overload and prevents increased blood viscosity.

5. Health maintenance

There are some lines of treatment that decreases the morbidity and mortality in children with sickle cell anemia, including:

1. Vaccination against capsulated organisms (e.g. Hib, Pneumococci, and meningococci).

2. Hydroxyurea and folic acid supplementation.

3. Oral penicillin prophylaxis in children less than 6 years.

4. Early detection and management of severe bacterial infections.

Hydroxyurea, by increasing HbF and thereby reducing sickling, decreases painful crises (by 50%) and decreases acute chest syndrome and transfusion requirements. The dose of hydroxyurea is variable and is adjusted to increase HbF.

Hydroxyurea is more effective in some patients if given with erythropoietin (40,000-60,000 units/week). However, hydroxyurea can cause neutropenia and thrombocytopenia. Hydroxyurea is also a teratogen and should not be given to females in the child-bearing period.

The screening for stroke in children with SCD is recommended to be done from age 2 to 16 years using transcranial Doppler flow studies. Risky children can get benefit from prophylactic, chronic partial exchange transfusions keeping HbS at < 30% of total Hb.

Erythropoietin use in patients with anemia not related to chemotherapy is associated with high incidence of venous thromboembolism and cardiopulmonary complications (as myocardial infarction); it is not useful in patients with sickle cell disease except possibly if given in combination with hydroxyurea.[23]

6. Novel medications

6.1.1. Omega-3 fatty acids

Omega-3 fatty acids are significantly reduced in SCD patients. In a single-center study conducted in Sudan, there was a randomized, placebo-controlled, double-blind design for studying the effect of omega-3 treatment on sickle cell anemia patients. One hundred and forty patients were monitored for 1 year, and it was found that omega-3 treatment leads to a decline in occlusive crises and blood transfusion. Treatment with omega-3 was well tolerated by the patients and needs further study. [24]

6.1. Prasugrel

It is a new thienopyridine P2Y12 ADP receptor antagonist, which inhibits ADP-mediated platelet activation and aggregation. Phase 2 randomized, double-blind, placebo controlled studies to examine safety were completed in adults. There were no hemorrhagic events requiring medical intervention in either study arm. Mean pain rates (percentage of days with pain) and intensity in the prasugrel arm were decreased compared with placebo. But, these results were not statistically significant. It was well tolerated and a phase 3 trial in children is registered. [25]

7. Prognosis

The life span of homozygous patients with SCD has gradually increased to > 50 years. Common causes of death are acute chest syndrome, recurrent infections, pulmonary embolism, infarction of a vital organ, and renal failure. [23]

8. Summary

Sickle cell disease is an inherited hemoglobinopathy affecting mainly the black races and leading to chronic hemolysis. The abnormal HbS found in homozygous patients changes the shape of RBCs to become sickle-shaped. These cells can occlude small blood vessels leading to ischemia and pain. The patients may be complicated by acute chest syndrome, sepsis, sequestration, and aplastic crises. Sickle cell disease is characterized by anemia and can be diagnosed by Hb electrophoresis. Blood transfusion may be needed for these patients.

Occlusive crises are treated mainly by pain killers. Hydroxyurea may decrease the frequency of these crises. Early management of bacterial infections and vaccination against capsulated organisms can prevent sepsis.

Author details

Ahmed K. Mansour*, Sohier Yahia, Rasha El-Ashry, Angi Alwakeel, Ahmad Darwish and Khalil Alrjjal

*Address all correspondence to: ak_mans@yahoo.com

Pediatric Hematology /Oncology Unit, Mansoura University Children`s Hospital, Mansoura University, Mansoura, Egypt

References

[1] National Heart Lung and Blood Institute. The management of SickleCell Disease. Publication #02-2117, 2002. www.nhlbi.nih.gov/health/prof/blood/sickle/sc mngt.pdf

[2] Perutz MF. Structure of haemoglobin. Brookhaven Symp Biol. 1960;13:165–183.

[3] Weatherall D, Clegg JB. The thalassaemia syndrome, 3rd ed. Oxford: Blackwell Science Ltd., 1981.

[4] Ferrone F, Nagel RL. Sickle hemoglobin polymerization. In: Steinberg MH, Forget BG, Higgs D, Nagel, editors. Disorders of hemoglobin: Genetics, pathophysiology, clinical management. Cambridge: Cambridge University Press, 2000.

[5] Kaul DK, Fabry ME, Nagel RL. Microvascular sites and characteristics of sickle cell adhesion to vascular endothelium in shear flow conditions: pathophysiological implications. Proc Natl Acad Sci USA. 1989;86:3356–3360.

[6] Steinberg MH, Forget BG, Higgs D, Nagel, editors. Disorders of hemoglobin: Genetics, pathophysiology, clinical management. Cambridge: Cambridge University Press, 2000.

[7] Lazarus, Hillard M, Schmaier, Alvin H. *Concise Guide to Hematology.* Wiley-Blackwell, 2011 p. 18. ISBN 1-4051-9666-1.

[8] How Does Sickle Cell Cause Disease? http://sickle.bwh.harvard.edu/scd background.html [Accessed 27 November 2010].

[9] Sickle Cell Anemia: eMedicine Emergency Medicine. http://emedicine.medscape.com/article/205926-overview [Accessed 27 November 2010].

[10] Caughey WS. Biochemical and clinical aspects of hemoglobin abnormalities. New York: Academic Press, 1978.

[11] Diwani M. Erythroblastic anaemia with bone changes in Egyptian children.Possibly Cooleys anaemia. Arch Dis Child. 1944;19:163–168.

[12] Abbasy AS. Sickle cell anemia; first case reported from Egypt. Blood. 1951;6:555–558.

[13] Lehmann H. Variations in human haemoglobin synthesis and factors governing their inheritance. Br Med Bull. 1959;15:40–46.

[14] El-Hazmi MAF, Warsy AS. Hemoglobinopathies in Arab countries. In: Teebi AS, Farag TL, editors. Genetic disorders among Arab populations. New York: Oxford University Press, 1997, pp. 83–110.

[15] Essential Haematology, edition 6, AV Hoffbrand, JE Petit, and PAH Moss.

[16] Ballas SK, Lieff S, Benjamin LJ, et al. Definitions of the phenotypic manifestations of sickle cell disease. Am J Hematol 2010;85:6–13

[17] Clarke GM, Higgins TN. Laboratory investigation of hemoglobinopathies and thalassemias: review and update. Clin. Chem. 2000;46 (8 Pt 2): 1284–1290. PMID 10926923.

[18] BestBets: Does routine urinalysis and chest radiography detect occult bacterial infection in sickle cell patients presenting to the accident and emergency department with painful crisis? http://www.bestbets.org/bets/bet.php?id=1102. [Accessed 27 November 2010].

[19] Bellet PS, Kalinyak KA, Shukla R, Gelfand MJ, Rucknagel DL. Incentive spirometry to prevent acute pulmonary complications in sickle cell diseases. N Engl J Med 1995;333:699–703.

[20] Ohene-Frempong K, Weiner SJ, Sleeper LA et al. Cerebrovascular accidents in SCD: rates and risk factors. Blood 1998;91:288–294.

[21] Gaston MH, Verter JI. Woods G, et al. Prophylaxis with oral penicillin in children with sickle cell anemia. A randomized trial. N Engl J Med 1986;314(25):1593–1599.

[22] Thachil J. Sickle cell disease management. *Haematology in Critical Care: a practical handbook*, 1st edn. John Wiley & Sons, Ltd, 2014.

[23] Sickle Cell Disease: Anemias caused by hemolysis: Merck Manual Professional. 2014. http://www.merckmanuals.com/professional/hematologyandoncology/anemiascausedbyhemolysis/sicklecelldisease.html?qt=sickle&alt=sh#v970306. [Accessed 29 September 2014].

[24] Daak AA, Ghebremeskel K, Hassan Z, et al. Effect of omega-3 (n-3) fatty acid supplementation in patients with sickle cell anemia: randomized, double-blind, placebo-controlled trial. Am J Clin Nutr. 2013;97(1):37–44.

[25] Wun T, Soulieres D, Frelinger AL, et al. A double-blind, randomized, multicenter phase 2 study of prasugrel versus placebo in adult patients with sickle cell disease. J Hematol Oncol. 2013;6(1):17.

Chapter 4

Interaction between Erythropoiesis and Iron Metabolism in Human β-thalassemia - Recent Advances and New Therapeutic Approaches

Nadia Maria Sposi

Additional information is available at the end of the chapter

http://dx.doi.org/10.5772/61716

Abstract

For its frequency and severity β-thalassemia represents a significant health problem in various areas of the world. Progressive iron overload is a common complication of hemoglobinopathies and represents a major cause of morbidity and premature mortality in patients with β-thalassemia.The discovery of hepcidin and its role in iron homeostasis has revolutionized our understanding of the pathogenesis of iron overload and iron-restricted anemias, stimulating the development of new diagnostic and therapeutic modalities for these disorders. However, little is known about the relationship among ineffective erythropoiesis, the role of iron-regulatory genes, and tissue iron distribution in β-thalassemia. The chapter describes evidences for these relationships and discusses how recent discoveries on iron metabolism and erythropoiesis could lead to new therapeutic approaches and better clinical care of these diseases.

Keywords: Thalassemia, Erythropoiesis, Iron Metabolism, Hepcidin, Ferroportin

1. Introduction

In recent years there has been important advancement in our knowledge of iron metabolism regulation that also has implications for understanding the pathophysiology of some human disorders such as beta-thalassemia (β-thalassemia) and other overload diseases. Progressive iron overload has become a major cause of morbidity and premature mortality in patients with β-thalassemia. However, little is known about the relationship among ineffective erythropoiesis, the role of iron-regulatory genes, and tissue iron distribution in β-thalassemia. Our understanding of the pathogenesis of iron-restricted anemias and iron overload has been revolutionized by the discovery of hepcidin and its role in iron homeostasis, stimulating the development of new diagnostic and therapeutic modalities for these disorders. Further work is required to understand the mechanisms of hepcidin regulation by iron and erythroid activity and to understand the structure, the transport function and the complex regulation of the hepcidin receptor ferroportin. The chapter describes evidences for these relationships and discusses how recent discoveries on iron metabolism and erythropoiesis could lead to new therapeutic approaches and better clinical care of these diseases, thereby yelding a much better quality of life for patients suffering from iron disorders and anemias.

2. Overall view on β-thalassemia

β-thalassemias are a group of hereditary blood disorders characterized by the reduced (β^{+} or β^{++}) or absent (β^{0}) synthesis of the β-globin chains of the hemoglobin (Hb) tetramer. The term thalassemia is derived from the Greek words *thalassa* (sea) and *haima* (blood) and is one of the most common autosomal recessive disorders worldwide. β-thalassemia is prevalent in Mediterranean countries, the Middle East, Central Asia, Far East, as well as countries along the Americas (Fig.1). The highest incidences are reported in Cyprus (14%), Sardinia (12%) and South-East Asia [1–3]. The high gene frequency of β-thalassemia in these regions is most likely related to the selective pressure from Plasmodium falciparum malaria [1–2]. Carriers of β-thalassemia are indeed relatively protected against the invasion of Plasmodium falciparum. However, because of population migration and intermarriage between different ethnic groups, β-thalassemia is, at present, also common in Northern Europe, North and South America,the Caribbean and Australia [4]. The inability to synthesize β-globin chains results in an excess of α-globin chains that precipitate in red cell precursors and cause abnormal cell maturation and their premature destruction in the bone marrow (ineffective erythropoiesis). Red cells that survive to reach the peripheral circulation are prematurely destroyed in the spleen. The clinical manifestations of β-thalassemia are extremely diverse, spanning a broad spectrum from the transfusion-dependent state of thalassemia major (TM) to the asymptomatic state of heterozygous carriers for β° or β^{+} (thalassemia trait).

β-thalassemias can be classificated into:

- Thalassemia major
- Thalassemia intermedia
- Thalassemia minor

β-thalassemia with associated Hb anomalies:

- Hb C/β-thalassemia
- Hb E/β-thalassemia
- Hb S/β-thalassemia

http://dx.doi.org/10.5772/61716

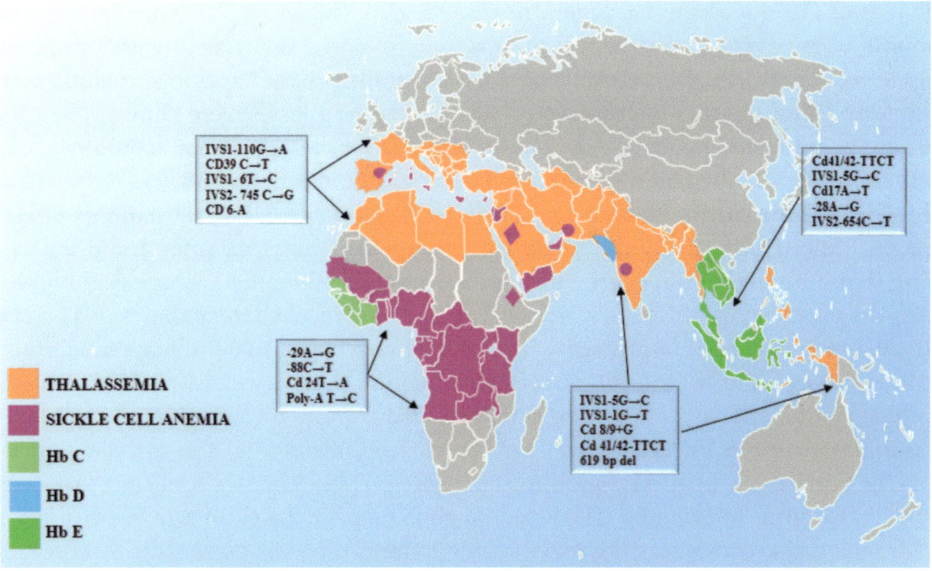

Figure 1. Thalassemia distribution and most common β-thalassemia mutations in different countries.

Hereditary persistence of fetal Hb and β-thalassemias

Autosomal dominant forms

β-thalassemia associated with other manifestations:

- β-thalassemia- tricothiodystrophy
- x-linked thrombocytopenia with thalassemia

Many different mutations cause β-thalassemia. They are inherited in a multitude of genetic combinations responsible for a heterogeneous group of clinical syndromes. Thalassemia minor, also known as β-thalassemia trait or heterozygous β-thalassemia, is caused by the presence of a single β-thalassemic mutation and a normal β-globin gene on the other chromosome. Microcytosis, hypochromia, increased HbA2 level and mild or minimal anemia are the characteristic hematological features of beta-thalassemia carriers. The β-thalassemia carrier state is clinically asymptomatic and needs no specific treatment. Thalassemia major, also known as Cooley's anemia or homozygous β-thalassemia, is a clinically severe disorder that results from the inheritance of two β-thalassemia alleles, one on each copy of chromosome 11. Patients have a severe microcytic and hypochromic anemia, associated with increased number of red blood cells and low mean corpuscular volume (MCV) and mean corpuscular Hb (MCH). Peripheral blood smear shows, in addition to microcytosis and hypochromia, anisocytosis, poikilocytosis and nucleated red blood cells (e.g., erythroblasts) [4]. The anemia of thalassemia major is so severe that chronic blood transfusions are usually required. Repeated transfusions and increased iron absorption lead to iron deposition in many organs (liver, endocrine tissues, heart) and ultimately death unless chelation therapy is used [5]. Hemoglobin analysis shows mainly HbF plus a small amount of HbA_2 in β^0 homozygotes, but insufficient to compensate for the loss of HbA, and the Hb level remains <5 g/dL [5]. Most β^+ homozygotes and $\beta^+\beta^0$ compound heterozygotes also have thalassemia major. HbF remains the predominant hemoglobin but with variable amounts of HbA depending on the specific β^+ thalassemia allele [5]. The term β-thalassemia intermedia (TI) is applied to a less severe clinical phenotype in which significant anemia occurs but chronic transfusion therapy is not absolutely required. Patients show a markedly heterogeneous hematological picture, ranging in severity from that of the β-thalassemia carrier state to that of thalassemia major [4]. Most patients affected by thalassemia intermedia are homozygotes or compound heterozygotes for β-thalassemia, meaning that both β-globin loci are affected. Less commonly, only a single β-globin locus is affected, the other being completely normal. The mild clinical characteristics of TI compared with thalassemia major result primarily from the inheritance of two β-thalassemia mutations, one mild and one severe; the inheritance of two mild mutations or, occasionally, the inheritance of complex combinations, such as two β-thalassemia mutations co-inherited with heterozygous α-thalassemia. In this last form, known as αβ-thalassemia, the α-thalassemia allele reduces the burden of unpaired α-globin chains [6–9]. Table 1 shows some of the commonest causes of thalassemia intermedia. The β-globin gene maps in the short arm of chromosome 11 an 80 Kb region also containing the δ globin gene, the embryonic ε gene, the fetal Aγ and Gγ gene [4]. The five functional globin genes are arranged in the order of their developmental expression (Fig 2) [4]. The β-globin gene is regulated by an adjacent 5′ promoter in which a Tata, CAAT and duplicated CACC boxes are located [4]. A major regulatory region, containing also a strong enhancer, maps 50 Kb from the β-globin gene. This locus control region (LCR) contains four (HS-1 to HS-4) erythroid specific DNAse hypersensitive sites (HS_S) containing a variety of binding sites for erythroid transcription factors [4,10–11]. The LCR together with the proximal cis-element transcription factors controls the developmental stage specific expression of genes: from ε to γ, and from γ to β and δ during development from embryo to adult. Very early in gestation there is a switch from ε to γ-globin production. The fetal hemoglobin (HbF) reaches a plateau after 10– weeks and remains high until 2– years after birth, when it begins to decrease to 0.5–1 % of total hemoglobin in adult red blood cells. The β-globin chain synthesis starts at 30–35– weeks of gestation contributing at this time to 10% of the total hemoglobin. After birth it increases to 97 % forming the adult hemoglobin HbA. The other type of adult hemoglobin is the HbA_2 formed by δ chains whose synthesis begins at the 7 th– month of gestation reaching 2–3% in adult life (Fig 2) [12]. Forms of β-thalassemia arise from mutations that affect every step in the pathway of globin gene expression: transcription, processing of the mRNA precursor, translation of mature mRNA, and post-translational integrity of the β-polipeptide chain [13]. Over 200 different thalassemia alleles of the β-globin gene have been reported; the vast majority are caused by point mutations within the gene or its immediate flanking sequences. The distribution of alleles is highly variable from one population to another but within each population there are only a few alleles that are common (Fig 1) [5]. While most alleles behave as Mendelian recessives, there are variants that cause a disease phenotype even when present in a single copy. These act in a dominant negative fashion and are referred to as dominantly inherited β-thalassemias [5]. Conditions with HbF production high enough to give good compensation are known as hereditary persistence of foetal hemoglobin (HPFH) and homozygotes are clinically unaffected while compound heterozygotes with β-thalassemia are very mild [5]. Fetal hemoglobin is a much more common and major modifier of disease severity in individuals with β-thalassemia. In normal individuals only 5-8% of red cells, called F cells, contains HbF,amounting to 5-20% of the total hemoglobin in those cells [14,15]. In the context of a severe deficiency of β-globin synthesis, even the low levels of γ-globin in F cells reduce the relative excess of a α -globin and provide a potent selective survival advantage for cells making HbF in the context of the ineffective erythropoiesis characteristic of the most severe forms of β-thalassemia [14]. Some β-thalassemia mutations increase " per se" the γ-globin gene synthesis, i.e. deletion and non deletion δβ-thalassemia or deletions of the 5′ region of the beta-globin gene. Also mutations associated with deletion and non-deletion HPFH linked to the β-globin gene cluster are characterized by increasing HbF production. Recently, the genome-wide association studies (GWAS) revealed genetic elements not linked to the β-globin gene cluster, able to modify the severity of the homozygous β^0- thalassemia. In particular, two new regulatory pathways leading to increased γ-globin expression have been identified, i.e. BCL11A and HBS1L-MYB. Both seem to act directly or indirectly affecting the production of repressor proteins that specifically target the γ-globin genes [16]. The clinical phenotype of homozygous β-thalassemia may also be modified by co-inheritance of other genetic variants mapping outside the globin clusters:. the presence of $(TA)_7$ polymorphism in the promoter region of the uridine diphosphate-glucuronosyltransferase gene is a risk factor for the development of cholelitiasis in thalassemia major and intermedia patients; the apolipoprotein E ε4 allele and some HLA haplotypes, which seem to be genetic risk factors for left ventricular failure in homozygous beta-thalassemia; a polymorphism in glutathione-S transferase M1 gene has been associated with an increased risk of heart iron overload in thalassemia major [1]. The expression of β-globin genes is also affected by point mutations belonging to three different categories: mutations of promoter and 5'UTR lead to defective β-gene transcription; mutations of splice-junction and 3'UTR affect mRNA processing; and non-sense, frameshift, and initiation codon mutations result in abnormal mRNA translation. Phatophysiology of β-thalassemia can be summarized as follows: the reduced amount or absence of β-globin chains result in a relative excess of unbound α-globin chains that precipitate in erythroid precursors in the bone marrow. Aggregation, denaturation and degradation of these chains lead to the formation of insoluble precipitates as well as hemichromes, which damage cell membranes leading to their premature death and hence to ineffective erythropoiesis. Red cells hemolysis within the circulation and membrane binding of IgG and C3 causes loss of red cells in the spleen. The resulting anemia leads to diminished tissue oxygenation, an increase in erythropoietin levels and bone marrow stimulation and expansion causing skeletal deformities and osteopenia. Substances released from damaged red cells increase iron absorption contributing to iron overload [14]. Diagnosis of β-thalassemia is based on hematologic and molecular genetic testing. Differential diagnosis is usually straightforward but may include genetic sideroblastic anemias, congenital dyserythropoietic anemias and other conditions with high levels of HbF. Genetic counseling is recommended and prenatal diagnosis may be offered. Prognosis of thalassemia minor subjects is excellent. Individuals with thalassemia intermedia may require splenectomy, folic acid supplementation, treatment of extramedullary erythropoietic masses and leg ulcers, prevention and therapy of thromboembolic events. Patients with thalassemia intermedia who do not usually have severe hemosiderosis are less prone to cardiac problems [1,17]. The prognosis of β-thalassemia major was very grim before there was any treatment available. With no treatment, the natural history was for death by age five from infections and cachexia [1]. Treatment of thalassemia major includes regular RBC transfusions, iron chelation and management of secondary complications of iron overload. In some circumstances, spleen removal may be required. However, many transfusion-dependent patients continued to develop progressive accumulation of iron. This can lead to tissue damage and eventually death, particularly from cardiac disease. The introduction of new iron chelators and chelation regimes associated to the monitoring of myocardial siderosis and cardiac function have converted a once universally fatal disease to a chronic illness. Children treated with chelators since a very young age are expected to have an excellent long-term prognosis [18-19]. Stem cell transplantation is at present the only available definitive cure for patients with thalassemia major but still has a substantial risk of mortality and morbidity. Umbelical cord-blood transplantations have had limited success in the treatment of β-thalassemia because of the large numbers required to sustain hematopoiesis. LV-mediated gene therapy for the β-hemoglobinopathies is now entering early-phase clinical trials and offers great promise. Even if these approaches are successful, such molecular therapies are likely to be expensive and might not be immediately applied to most patients in low-income countries. Much evidence from clinical genetic studies shows that the induction of γ-globin chain synthesis by gene transduction or pharmacological agents would have substantial clinical benefits in patients with β-thalassemia [12,20–26]. However the results obtained have not been sufficiently encouraging to develop large-scale trials [12,24–26]. Furthermore, these agents have several effects, and how any of these drugs work to increase expression of HbF is not fully understood. Recently pre-clinical evidence of potentially new approaches to treating patients with TI and TM has been reported. The evidence for using Tf, hepcidin agonists and JAK2 inhibitors is discussed later in this chapter.

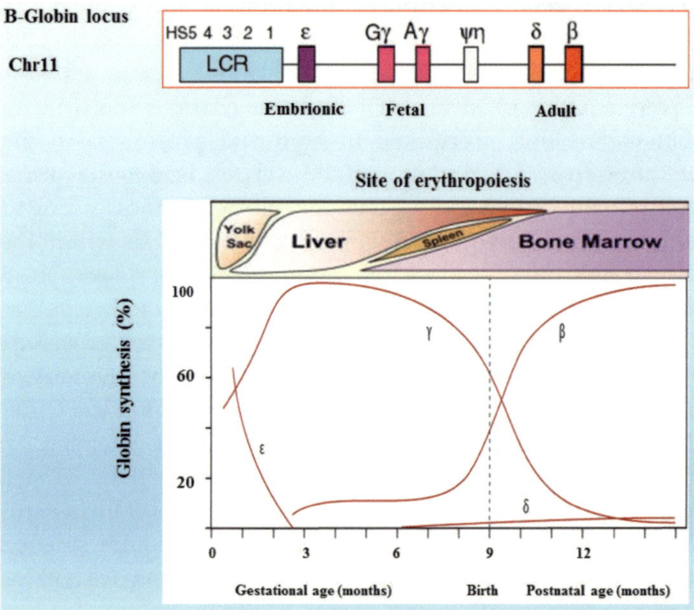

Figure 2. In the top panel, the organization of human β-globin locus is shown. Upstream DNase I hypersensitive sites (HS) within the locus control region (LCR) are displayed. The bottom panel shows the fetal-to-adult hemoglobin switch. This illustration depicts the normal timing of the developmental hemoglobin switches in humans. This figure is adapted from [4] and [12].

Mild deficit in β-chain production	· Homozygosity for silent or mild β-thal · Compound heterozygosity for severe and mild β-thal · HbE/ β-thal · Heterozygous β-thal with $\alpha\alpha\alpha$ or $\alpha\alpha\alpha\alpha$
Reduced α-chain excess	· Homozygous β° or β^+ thal with 2 or 3 α gene deletions · Homozygous β° or β^+ thal with non deletion α-thal · Homozygous β^+ thal with 1 or 2 α gene deletions
Increased γ-chain synthesis	· Homozygous (δβ)°-thal or (Aγδβ)°-thal · Homozygosity for Hb Lepore · Compound heterozygosity for Hb Lepore/β-thal · Compound heterozygosity for severe β-thal and HPFH
Dominant β-thalassemia	· Highly unstable β-chain variants · Bthal heterozygotes with third exon mutations

Table 1. The commonest causes of thalassemia intermedia

3. Overall view on erythropoiesis

The production of red blood cells, known as erythropoiesis, is a developmental system fundamentally under genetic control that involves differentiation of pluripotent hematopoietic stem cells (HSCs) and early multipotent progenitors (MPP) in erythroblasts and mature erythrocytes. Human erythroid differentiation is also regulated and modulated by the interaction of humoral, cellular and molecular processes [27–30]. The erythroid progenitor cell compartment contains the early erythroid progenitors (BFU-E, burst-forming units-erythroid), which differentiate into late colony-forming units erythroid (CFU-E) and proerythroblasts. BFU-E represent the earliest progenitors committed exclusively to erythroid maturation and a quiescent reserve because only 10% to 20% are in cycle at any given time. CFU-E is more differentiated than BFU-E and most of these progenitors (60–80%) are already in cycle. The earliest recognizable erythroid cells are the proerythroblasts, which differentiate in basophilic erythroblasts, followed by polychromatophilic and orthochromatic erythroblasts. After the last mitotic division, the inactive dense nucleus of the orthochromatic erythroblast is extruded and the resulting mature enucleated cell is a reticulocyte. Mature red blood cells are biconcave disks without mithocondria and other organelles, but with a very high concentration of hemoglobin able to bind and deliver O2 [29, for an exhaustive review see 31–37]. Fig. 3 schematically represents the pathway of erythropoiesis from progenitors to mature cells. The blood has a very important role in the functions of the organism from the earliest moments of its development, so that during embryonic life the various stages of the hematopoietic process alternate at different sites according to the different stages of development [38–39]. The embryonic → fetal hematopoiesis is characterized by three fundamental periods of activity progressively involving the yolk sac, liver and bone marrow. The first period, during which hematopoiesis is localized at the yolk sac, begins between the 14th and 19th days of embryonic life and continues until the completion of the 3rd month [38–39]. Starting from the third month, the second phase of hematopoiesis takes place in the liver where it reaches its maximum during the 3rd–4th month and remains active until a few weeks before birth, when the definitive hematopoiesis (third phase) is concentrated only in the bone marrow and it will continue throughout adult life [38]. In this system of hematopoietic differentiation four compartments may be identified: stem cells, the progenitors (cellular compartments), precursors, and mature elements of circulating blood (maturation compartments) [39]. Hematopoietic stem cells are characterized by the ability to self-renew (i.e., to generate other totipotent stem cells) and differentiate into hematopoietic progenitor cells. Stem cells also show the important property to remain for a long time in a state of quiescence during adult life [36–37,39–40]. Primitive progenitors are able to generate blast colonies (CFU-B), the progenitors of high proliferative potential (HPP-CFC, colony-forming cells that power high-proliferative), and finally the multipotent progenitors that are still capable of generating mixed colonies, belonging to the different types of hematopoietic differentiation: erythroid, granulocyte, monocyte, and megakaryocytic (the CFU-GEMM) [37,41–42]. Mature progenitors are committed to the differentiation towards a singular hematopoietic lineage and are functionally defined as early burst forming units (BFUs) or more differentiated colony forming units (CFUs): erythroid progenitors are BFU-E and CFU-E; granulocytic-macrophagic progenitors are CFU-GM, CFU-G and CFU-M; finally megakaryocitc progenitors are BFU-Mk and CFU-Mk [37,41–42]. The proliferation, maturation and differentiation of hematopoietic stem cells and progenitors are regulated by the interaction of several hematopoietic growth factors with specific membrane receptors and the consequent activation of the appropriate signal transduction pathways. These factors are also known as colony stimulating factors (CSFs), interleukins (ILs), or hemopoietins and are produced from accessory cells such as macrophages, lymphocytes, fibroblasts, and endothelial cells. They can be classified into three categories, depending on their mechanism of action during hemopoietic differentiation (Fig.3) [34,39]. In the first category are growth factors acting at the earliest stages of hematopoiesis, i.e. the stem cell factor (SCF) [43], FLT-3 ligand (FL) [44,45], the basic fibroblast growth factor (bFGF) [46,47], and interleukin-6 (IL-6) [48]. IL-3 and GM-CSF, growth factors acting as multilineage, belong to the second category and are able to stimulate primitive progenitors to proliferate and differentiate into all hematopoietic lineage [49]. The third category includes the unilineage growth factors acting on progenitors already committed and promoting the production of mature cells in the circulating blood, i.e. erythropoietin (EPO) [50–51], the granulocytic growth factor (G-CSF) [52], monocytic growth factor (M-CSF) [53], and thrombopoietin (TPO) [54]. During hematopoietic differentiation, the maintenance of iron homeostasis is essential for erythrocytes and macrophages. Erythroid cells need to incorporate very high amounts of iron to support the continued synthesis of heme and hemoglobin, while the macrophage cells play a key role in the storage and recycling of iron [29,39,55–56]. During the differentiation of erythroid progenitors towards mature red cells the following morphologically recognizable stages can be distinguished: 1) the earlier stage of proerythroblast, that presents a nucleus relatively large in respect to the cytoplasm, and one or two nucleoli; 2) the more advanced basophilic erythroblast, characterized by a reduced cellular diameter, a nuclear volume reduced more rapidly than the cytoplasm, and a cytoplasm uniformly basophilic; 3) the polychromatophilic erythroblast, that shows the initial condensation of the nucleus, nucleoli no longer visible and the cytoplasm with acidophilic areas; 4) the orthochromatic erythroblast, with a nucleus:cytoplasm ratio of approximately 1:4, nucleus darker and subject to pyknotic degeneration, and cytoplasm slightly pink as a consequence of the progressive increase in hemoglobin concentration; and finally 5) the reticulocyte that has lost its nucleus and, through the complete

http://dx.doi.org/10.5772/61716

degradation of ribosomes and mitochondria, proceeds to the transformation in mature erythrocyte [34,37,39,42,57–58]. In adult mammalian bone marrow erythroblasts are always associated with the erythroblastic islets that represent the drive amplification stage anatomy of erythropoiesis and consists of 1 or 2 histiocytic crown cells surrounded by erythroblasts at all stages of maturation. The histiocytes have thin cytoplasmic extensions that insert between erythroblasts suggesting that factors of nutrition can be provided by the histiocytic cell, centrally located, to the peripheral maturing erythroblasts [37,39,42]. The most important factor involved in the control of erythropoiesis is erythropoietin, but other substances, particularly hormones, contribute to the regulation of this process [59]. Transferrin comes out from the bone marrow sinusoids using ample fenestrature exits, and binds to surface receptors carried by erythroblasts. The iron transferred from transferrin and transported to the mitochondria is reduced from Fe^{3+} to Fe^{2+} and then inserted into protoporphyrin IX by tetrapyrroles heme synthetase (Heme Synthetase HS) for the synthesis of heme [39,55–56,59]. The reticuloendothelial system is a functional unit that includes cells having heterogeneous histologically different identities and a widespread distribution throughout the body, which share the common property of phagocytic activity, e.g. endothelial cells of blood capillaries of liver, spleen, bone marrow and lymph-nodes, tissue and circulating macrophages [59–60].The reticuloendothelial system is the most important source of iron that enters the blood compartment. The flow of iron from the reticuloendothelial plasma is unidirectional, as the reticuloendothelial cells are not able to pick up the metal from transferrin, but receive only hemoglobin or ferritin iron [59–60]. Senescent erythrocytes at the end of their life (approximately 120–days) are phagocytized by endothelial cells and represent the largest source of iron entering the reticuloendothelial system. About 85% of the iron that enters the reticuloendothelial cells is promptly transferred to plasma transferrin and the remaining 15% is stored as intracellular ferritin, and transferred to plasma much more slowly [39,42,59–60]. The production of red blood cells is regulated by a complex network of transcription factors, among which GATA-1 is considered the master gene of erythropoiesis. GATA-1 positively regulates specific erythroid genes such as erythropoietin receptor (EpoR), glycophorin (GpA), and globin chains and, together with the transcription factor STAT5, induces the expression of the antiapoptotic protein Bcl-xL (Fig.3 and Table 2) [61–63]. The program of erythroid proliferation and differentiation must be positively and negatively regulated to ensure a continuous but tightly controlled production of red blood cells. Erythropoiesis is positively controlled by the combined effect of two major cytokinesis, SCF and Epo. SCF is produced by stromal cells and exerts its effects on erythroid cells mainly during the early and late stages of differentiation of erythroid progenitors, and may act also on immature erythroid precursors. Epo is responsible for the finely tuned homeostatic control of erythrocyte numbers by tissue oxygenation. Epo exerts its effect by stimulating Epo-R. The binding of Epo with the EpoR induces a conformational change that activates the pre-bound, cytoplasmic tyrosine kinase JAK2. The activation of JAK2 induces multiple signaling pathways involving P13 kinase, Akt and STAT5, which prevent apoptosis, supporting erythroid progenitors proliferation and differentiation (Fig.3) [63–66]. However, a negative control of erythropoiesis is clearly required at several levels to avoid overproduction of erythroid cells and polycythemia, which may lead to hyperviscosity and ultimately to thrombosis. The negative regulation is mainly due to apoptosis, a fundamental cellular mechanism allowing clearance of unneeded or potentially dangerous cells. Caspases appear to play a critical role in erythroid apoptotic programs. Caspases belong to a family of cysteine-dependent and aspartate-specific proteases and, in particular, two classes are described: initiators (caspase-8 and –9) and effectors (caspase-3 and –7). Caspase-8 is activated by the death receptor pathway and caspase-9 by events causing intracellular damages and alterations in mitochondrial membrane potential. Activated caspase –8 and caspase –9 then activate effectors such as caspase –3 that cleaves GATA-1, Tal-1, and proteins involved in cytoplasm, nucleus, and DNA integrity, which allow the cell death program to occur. Death receptors of the TNF receptor (TNF-R) superfamilies (Fas-L, TNF-α, TRAIL) activate the extrinsic apoptotic pathway. Some studies suggest the existence of a negative regulatory feedback operating at low Epo level in a paracrine pathway. Briefly the control of mature red blood cell production may be summarized as follow: at low doses of Epo, cells die by apoptosis, at intermediate doses, cells are arrested in their maturation or enter a program of apoptosis, depending on the number of mature erythroblasts in the bone marrow, and at high doses of Epo, erythroid progenitors and precursors pursue their maturation independently of the number of mature erythroid precursors [63,67–68]. In summary, the emerging picture is that certain genes, such as SCL, are absolutely required for hematopoietic development, whereas others, such as GATA- 2, c-Myb, CBF and some downstream signal transducing molecules, such as Jack 2 and STAT5, are responsible for expansion and maintenance of a normal pool of fetal liver and adult hematopoietic progenitors. The participation of many of these molecules in multicomponent molecular complexes with protein/protein and protein/DNA interactions (e.g., LMO2/Lmbd1/SCL/GATA), during the early, proliferative stages of hematopoiesis may underlie their role in the proliferation and maintenance of immature progenitor/precursor pools in erythropoiesis [69]. Other genes such as GATA1, its partner FOG1, and EKLF are necessary to direct high levels of function of erythroid-specific genes in cells already committed to terminal differentiation. Thus, a hierarchical requirement in the expression of specific regulators during early versus late erythroid differentiation or during embryonic versus fetal liver/adult erythropoiesis is established.

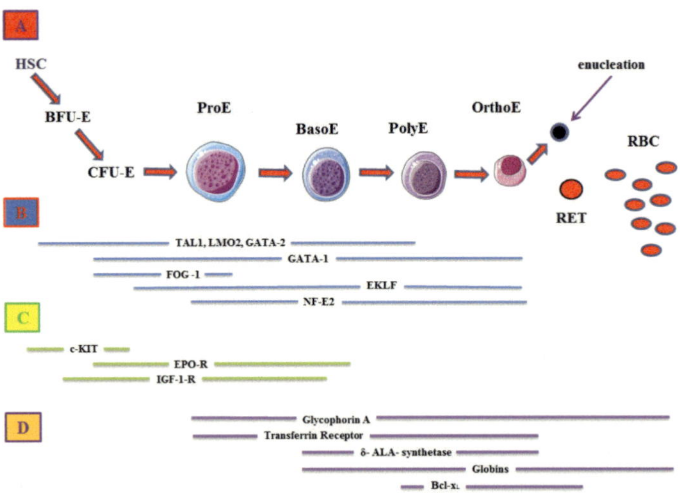

Figure 3. A) Pathway of the erythropoiesis from progenitors to mature cells. Different stages are indicated: hematopoietic stem cell (HSC), burst-forming unit erythroid (BFU-E), colony-forming unit erythroid (CFU-E), proerythroblast (ProE), basophylic (BasoE), polychromatic (PolyE), and orthochromatic erythroblast (OrthoE). **B)** Erythroid transcrip-

tion factors: basic helix-loop-helix factor (TAL1); Lim-domain partner of TAL1 (LMO2); zinc finger factors that bind GATA sequences (GATA-1, GATA-2); GATA-1 partner, friend of GATA (FOG); erythroid Kruppel-like factor (EKLF) and p45NF-E2 (NF-E2). **C)** Receptors for hematopoietic growth factors: stem cell factor-receptor/c-kit; erythropoietin receptor (EPO-R) and insulin-like growth factor-1 receptor (IGF-1-R). **D)** Proteins related to erythrocyte structure and function. Modified by [39] and [32].

Trans-acting factor	Binding motif	Role in hematopoiesis	Target genes	Phenotype of gene inactivation	Human pathology
GATA-1	(A/T) GATA (A/G)	↑ Erythroid differentiation	Globin, erithroid, specific membrane proteins, GATA-1, GATA-2	Anemia and trombocytopenia	X-linked thalassemia/ trombocytopenia
GATA-2	(A/T) GATA (A/G)	↑ Proliferation ↓ Differentiation	GATA-1, GATA-2	No proliferation of immature progenitors	
FOG-1	None	GATA-1-cofactor		No erythroid maturation	
EKLF	CACC	Promotes terminal erythroid differentiation	Globin	Anaemia	β-thalassemia
SCL	CANNTG (E box)	Specification of hematopoiesis		Absence of prenatal hematopoiesis	Translocation in T-ALL
LM02	Lim domain			Absence of hematopoiesis	T-CELL acute lymphocytic leukemia
Myb	(T/C) AAC (G/T) G	↓ Definitive erythropoiesis		Block in definitive erythropoiesis	
STAT 5	GAS	Antiapoptotic effect at level of erythroid precursors	BCL-XL	Anemia due to apoptosis of erythroid progenitors	
NFE 2	TGAGTCA	Promotes terminal erythroid differentiation in vitro	Enzyme of the haem biosynthetic pathway,globin	trombocytopenia	

Table 2. Major transcription factors/signaling molecules involved in the control of erythropoiesis. DNA-binding sites and known target genes of the indicated transcription factors together with the phenotype of their gene inactivation in mice and the human pathologies associated with gene mutations are shown.

4. Iron metabolism and erythropoiesis

Iron plays a pivotal role in cell survival and proliferation by regulating enzymatic activity and oxidation-reduction reactions. It is essential primarily for ensuring the transport of oxygen and for the catalysis of reactions involved in electron transfer, nitrogen fixation and DNA synthesis, but it is also toxic due to its capacity to react with oxygen and catalyze the production of reactive oxygen species. In solution, iron can exist in two states of oxidation, Fe (II) and Fe (III), and is very poorly soluble at physiological pH, especially when it is in the oxidized form Fe (III). Living organisms have thus developed many proteins to carry iron in biological fluids and transport it through cellular membranes, and to store it in a non-toxic and easily mobilizable form [70–72]. Erythropoiesis and iron metabolism are processes closely linked to each other. The large majority of iron in our body is utilized by the erythropoietic system to generate functionally active hemoglobin molecules, which are harbored in the red blood cells. It is estimated that 1800 mg of iron in our body is present in red blood cells, 300 mg in the bone marrow and 600 mg in the reticuloendothelial macrophages of the spleen [71], accounting for more than 60% of total body iron. Approximately 10% is present in muscle fibers (in myoglobin) and other tissues (in enzymes and cytochromes) and the remaining body iron is stored in the liver. The normal diet contains 15–20 mg of iron, and the body absorbs 1–2 mg/d of dietary iron. This is balanced with losses via sloughed intestinal mucosal cells, menstruation and other blood losses. Therefore, internal turnover of iron is essential to meet the bone marrow requirements for erythropoiesis (20–30 mg/d) (Fig. 4) [73–75]. This massive utilization of iron by the erythropoietic system requires the presence of finely tuned regulatory systems that allow storage, mobilization and traffic of iron and at the same time prevent toxicity due to highly reactive iron ions. Because there are no physiologically regulated means of iron excretion, dietary iron absorption is highly regulated primarily at the level of duodenal enterocytes. Other important regulatory sites are the liver and the spleen. Hepatocytes and Kuppfer cells can store large quantities of iron, while iron from senescent red blood cells is recycled from macrophages in the spleen. All three compartments are of pivotal importance for erythropoiesis since they control the bioavailability of iron to erythroid progenitors, and all of them respond to hepcidin, the master regulator of iron metabolism [76]. A summary of proteins involved in iron homeostasis, as well as their most frequently used acronyms, is given in Table 3 and Table 4. Transferrin is the main plasma iron transporter that binds two molecules of ferric iron (Fe3+). At the systemic level, transferrin satuaration is the main iron sensor and plays a role in controlling the levels of the iron-regulatory peptide hepcidin [77]. Transferrin is usually between 20 and 30% satured with iron. At the cellular level we known two common mechanisms that can be applied to most of the proteins involved in iron metabolism regulation. First, iron- regulatory proteins 1 (IRP1) and 2 (IRP2) bind to iron-response elements (IREs) in the untranslated regions (UTRs) of mRNA encoding protein involved in cellular iron uptake, storage, and export. IRP1 and IRP2 bind to IREs under conditions of low iron, and they dissociate from IREs in high-iron states [77–78]. If the IRE is in 3'UTR, IRP binding stabilizes the mRNA, prevents degradation, and increases protein production. If the IRE is in the 5'UTR, mRNA translation is inihibited. There are over 35 mRNAs, including hypoxia-inducible factor 2α, that have an IRE and are responsive to iron. The second general mechanism imparts tissue-specific sensitivity to iron balance by modulation of the proportion of iron-sensitive and iron-insensitive mRNAs. This means that one variant responds to iron levels and one does not. The ratio of IRE to non-IRE differs in different tissues, resulting in differences in responsiveness to iron and differences in loading [77]. In specialized cell types, alternatively spliced non-IRE-containing isoforms of ferroportin [34] and DMT1 [79] mRNAs bypass post-transcriptional regulation by IRPs. Under normal circumstances, dietary ferric iron is reduced by cytochrome B to ferrous iron (Fe 2+) at the apical brush border of duodenal enterocytes and transported into the cell by DMT1. DMT1 expression is highest at the duodenum and decreases towards the colon. Dietary heme iron is absorbed into the enterocyte via the heme carrier protein-1 Inside the enterocyte, heme is degraded by heme oxygenase and iron is released into the cytosol. The free iron is stored in the cells by ferritin or exported to the plasma by FPN1 [77,80–81]. Exported iron is loaded onto transferrin. Before the loading of transferrin, ferrous iron is oxidized to Fe 3+ by hephaestin. Cells can then take up transferrin-bound iron via transferrin receptor 1 (Tfr1, aka CD71). Erythroblasts, the major iron consuming cells in the organism, mainly take up transferrin-bound iron via transferrin receptor 1 (TfR1). Iron release takes place in vesicles of low pH. Ferric iron is reduced to ferrous iron by Steap3 and subsequently exported into the cytosol via DMT1, while transferrin and TfR1 recycle to the surface. The bulk of intracellular iron in erythroblasts is used for hemoglobin synthesis, where mitochondria are indispensable for heme production. Excess heme is either exported via FLVCR or catabolized via the HO-1 pathway [39,82]. As the intake of nutritional iron is not sufficient to cover the daily iron necessity of erythropoiesis, iron recycling is necessary. Macrophages exert a crucial role in iron recycling, phagocytosing senescent erythrocytes, and releasing accumulated iron back into the circulation in a regulated manner, thus enabling iron recycling [82]. Phagocytosed erythrocytes are broken up in lysosomes, and heme-bound iron is released via HO-1. When body iron levels are low, storage iron re-enters the circulation. Ferroportin again functions as the only known iron exporter, and another plasma copper-containing ferroxidase coeruloplasmina converts ferrous into ferric iron before its loading onto transferrin [82]. Similar to reticuloendothelial cells, hepatocytes are an important site of iron storage in the form of ferritin. Most important, hepatocytes serve a central role in iron homeostasis as the site of regulated production of the hormone hepcidin. Hepcidin functions as the "hypoferremia hormone" by down-regulating the ferroportin-mediated release of iron into the circulation [83]. The consequent iron retention in duodenal enterocytes decreases dietary iron absorption and the iron retention in reticuloendothelial macrophages decreases iron turnover. Hepatocellular hepcidin production is regulated by signals reflecting inflammation, iron status, erythropoietic activity, and oxygen tension [83]. Major pathways of iron traffic between cells and tissues are indicated in Fig. 4.

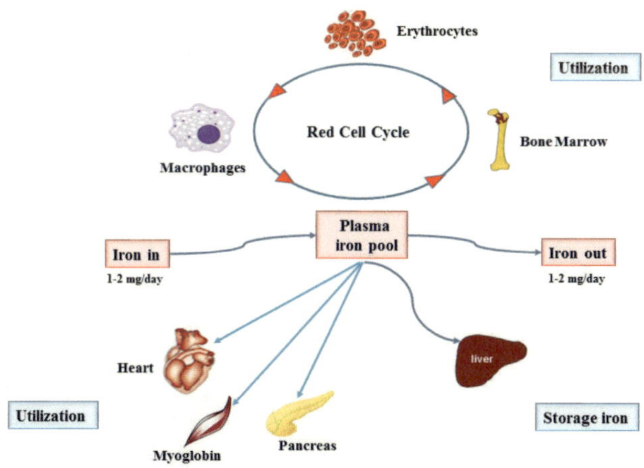

Figure 4. Major pathways of iron traffic between cells and tissues.

Protein name	Acronyms	Funcion in iron metabolism	Localization
Iron aquisition			
Transferrin	Tf	Plasma iron transfer	Plasma
Transferrin receptor 1	TfR1	Internalization of holo-Tf	Ubiquitously expressed
Six transmembrane epithelial antigen of the prostate 3	STEAP3	Ferric reductase in the endosomes of erythroid cells	erythroblast
Divalent metal transporter 1	DMT1	Epithelial/endosomal transport of ferrous iron	Enterocyte (apical membrane)
Duodenal cytochrome b	Dcytb	Apical membrane ferric reductase of enterocytes	Enterocyte (apical membrane)
Heme oxygenase 1	HO-1	Degradation of hemoglobin for Fe^{2+} release	Enterocyte
Ferritin	Ft	Cellular iron storage and uptake	Enterocyte, erythroblast , macrophage, hepatocyte, myocytes and cardiomyocytes
Intracellular iron transport			
Mitoferrin 1/2	MFRN 1/2	Import of ferrous iron to mitochondria	Erythroblast (mitochondria)
Iron efflux			
Ferroportin	FPN1	Export of ferrous iron	Enterocyte (basolateral membrane) Macrophages, hepatocytes, Erythroid cells
Hephaestin	HEPH	Membrane-bound ferroxidase	Enterocyte (basolateral)
Ceruloplasmin	CP	Plasma ferroxidase	macrophage
Feline leukemia virus, subgroup C, receptor	FLVCR	Heme export	Erythroblast

Table 3. Main proteins involved in iron homeostasis

PROTEIN NAME Systemic iron metabolism	Acronyms	Function	Phenotype due to loss of function
Hepcidin	HEPC	Inhibition of ferroportin mediated efflux	Absent hepcidin expression. Iron overload at the level of liver and pancreas and at a lesser extent of heart (HH type2A)

PROTEIN NAME Systemic iron metabolism	Acronyms	Function	Phenotype due to loss of function
Bone morphogenetic protein 6	BMP6	Regulation of hepcidin expression in response to hepatic iron	Iron overload with decreased levels of hepcidin
Hemojuvelin	HJV	Enhancement of BMP signaling to hepcidin	Early onset severe iron overload with suppressed hepcidin expression (HH type2A)
Transferrin	Tf	Plasma iron transfer	Iron deficiency anemia with tissue iron overload
High Fe protein	HFE	Regulation of hepcidin expression by plasma iron	Iron overload with decreased levels of hepcidin (HH type 1)
Transferrin receptor 2	TfR2	Regulation of hepcidin expression by plasma iron	Iron overload with decreased levels of hepcidin (HH type 3)
SMAD 4	SMAD4	Signaling to hepcidin	Decreased hepcidin levels and iron overload
Matriptase-2	TMPRSS6	Proteolytic cleavage of Hjv	Macrocytic anemia with low iron stores and increased hepcidin
Neogenin	NEO	Regulation of Hjv	Hepatic iron overload
Cellular iron metabolism			
Iron regulatory protein 1	IRP 1	Post-transcriptional regulation of IRE-containing mRNAs	Not known
Iron regulatory protein 2	IRP 2	Post-transcriptional regulation of IRE-containing mRNAs	Misregulation of iron metabolism. Neurodegenerative disease due to iron accumulation in neurons and oligodendrocytes
F-box and leucine-rich repeat protein 5	FBXL 5	Iron-dependent ubiquitination and degradation of IRP 2	Embryonic lethality

Table 4. Main proteins involved in iron homeostasis regulation

5. Hepcidin: The link between erythropoiesis and iron regulation

In recent years, there has been important advancement in our understanding of iron metabolism, mainly as a result of the discovery of hepcidin, a key regulator of whole body iron homeostasis originally identified from urine as an antimicrobial peptide produced in the hepatocytes [84]. The aim of this chapter is beyond a complete picture of current knowledge on the hepcidin regulation, therefore I will focus only on those aspects that influence erythropoiesis directly or indirectly. Targeted deletion of the HAMP gene in mice or mutations in the human HAMP gene result in massive iron overload [85]. Conversely, high levels of hepcidin lead to decreased iron absorption and iron-restricted anemias. Therefore, hepcidin is a negative regulator of iron transport into plasma. Experimental data suggested that the hepcidin could be the regulator of iron absorption and recycling acting principally or solely by binding to ferroportin, the only known cellular iron exporter. The hepcidin-ferroportin interaction controls systemic iron homeostasis: hepcidin binds to ferroportin and induces its internalization and degradation. This mechanism regulates the distribution of iron in the body. When hepcidin levels are low, iron-exporting cells, including duodenal enterocytes, macrophages, and hepatocytes display abundant ferroportin and release iron into plasma. When hepcidin concentration increase, hepcidin binds to ferroportin, causing its phosphorylation, internalization, ubiquitylation, sorting through the multivesicular body pathway, and degradation in lysosomes, and iron is retained within cells in cytoplasmic ferritin [34,82,86–89]. Hepcidin is regulated at transcriptional level by different stimuli that can act as positive or negative regulators. The membrane isoform of hemojuvelin (HJV), transferrin receptor 2 (TfR2), IL-6, iron and the hemochromatosis protein HFE are all positive regulators of hepcidin transcription. On the contrary, hypoxia, anemia, iron deficiency, and erythroid expansion are all negative regulators of hepcidin expression. We know four major regulatory pathways that act through different signaling pathways to control the transcription of hepcidin, e.g. iron erythroid demand, hypoxia, iron store, and inflammation. Briefly, hepcidin transcription is activated by BMP-6 (Bone morphogenetic protein 6) via the SMAD pathway. Hemojuvelin (HJV) enhances the activity of the BMP receptor (BMP-R), while cleavage of HJV by TMPRSS6 suppresses this activity. Diferric Tf displaces the hemochromatosis protein (HFE) from the high-affinity transferrin receptor (TfR1) that associates with TfR2 enhancing signaling via BMP-R. Inflammatory cytokine IL-6 acts through its receptor (IL6-R) and the JAK2/STAT3 pathway to turn on hepcidin production. Growth differentiation factor 15 (GDF15), twisted gastrulation-1, erythroferrone (ERFE), hypoxia, and erythropoietin (Epo) reduce hepcidin transcription [89–93]. GDF15 is released by erythroid precursors and increased in hemoglobinopathies, e.g. thalassemia, congenital dyserythropoietic anemia type 1, and refractory anemia with ring sideroblasts. GDF15 is decreased post transfusion, in parallel with EPO and decreased marrow activity, resulting in increase in hepcidin. Twisted gastrulation (TWSG1), soluble HJV, and erythroferrone (ERFE) are other factors that are rapidly produced with increased erythroid activity and result in reduced hepcidin production. ERFE belongs to the C1q-tumor necrosis factor-related family of proteins. In response to EPO, ERFE is rapidly produced by erythroid precursors in the bone marrow and the spleen via signal transducer and activator of transcription 5 (STAT5). The canonical Janus kinase 2 (Jak2)/Stat5 signaling pathway is a known mediator of EPO response and stress erythropoiesis. Further work is necessary to confirm whether ERFE is the long-sought erythroid regulator responsible for hepcidin suppression and iron overload in patients with hereditary iron- loading anemia [92, 94–97]. Regulation of hepcidin production is shown in Fig.5

http://dx.doi.org/10.5772/61716

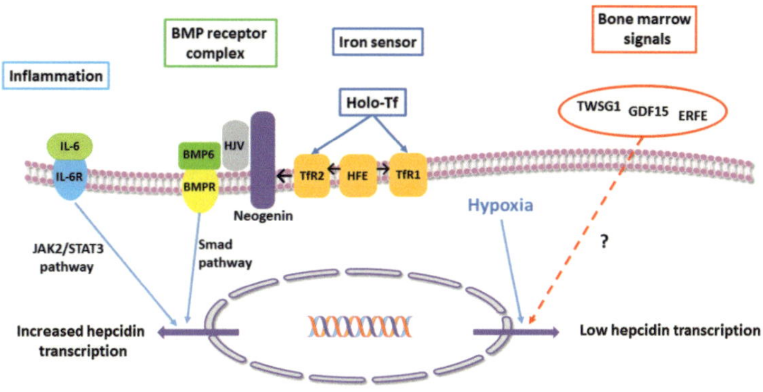

Figure 5. Iron-mediated regulation of hepcidin levels on hepatocytes.

6. Ineffective erythropoiesis and iron overload in β-thalassemia

In β-thalassemia the erythropoietic process is markedly altered and is referred to as ineffective erythropoiesis (IE). The lack or reduced synthesis of β-globin chains induces an excess of free α-globin chains within erythroid cells. Aggregation, denaturation, and degradation of these chains leads to the formation of insoluble precipitates that cause oxidative membrane damage within the red blood cell and developing erythroblasts [98]. In β-thalassemia the process of IE is accompanied by a massive iron overload, due to an increased rate of iron absorption by the gastrointestinal (GI) tract and to frequent blood transfusions. Nevertheless, iron overload occurs also in patients who have not received transfusions such as patients suffering from thalassemia intermedia [63,99]. In patients who are iron- overloaded, the capacity of serum transferrin to bind iron may be exceeded, which means that a non-transferrin-bound fraction of iron may circulate in the plasma. This unbound iron, which is carried in the iron storage protein ferritin, can promote the generation of free hydroxyl radicals, which propagate oxygen-related tissue damage. Additionally, insoluble iron complexes called hemosiderins may become deposited in body tissues causing toxicity and death. Cardiac failure is a major complication of iron overload. Iron deposition can cause myocarditis and cardiac fibrosis. There are a number of other possible complications of iron overload: excess iron deposition in the liver can lead to fibrosis/cirrhosis or cancer, and diabetes mellitus may occur as a result of beta-cell destruction secondary to iron overload in the pancreas. Excess iron overload in the pituitary may cause growth failure due to hypogonadism and infertility due to reduced gonadotropin levels [86,100–101]. If iron were a dominant regulator, patients with β-thalassemia should express very high levels of hepcidin in serum in order to decrease intestinal iron absorption. In contrast, the levels of hepcidin are very low in these patients, suggesting that the ineffective erythropoiesis alone is able to suppress the synthesis of hepcidin in spite of the presence of a severe iron overload [89,102–104]. Hepcidin deficiency develops as a result of a suppressive signal generated by the greatly expanded erythroid precursor population. This also leads to excessive iron absorption and the development of iron overload even in patients who are not transfused. Although the hepcidin suppression is partially relieved by erythrocyte transfusions, the transfusions themselves add large amounts of exogenous iron again leading to iron overload. The observation that serum from β-thalassemic patients inhibited hepcidin mRNA expression in the HepG2 cell line suggested the existence of a negative erythropoietic regulator of hepcidin expression [105]. The nature of this humoral factor is still uncharacterized, but may include one or more proteins during active erythropoiesis. One of this regulators could be the cytokine growth differentiation factor-15 (GDF15) because it was observed that serum from thalassemia patients suppressed hepcidin mRNA expression in primary human hepatocytes and depletion of GDF15 reversed the hepcidin expression. GDF15 is a divergent member of the transforming growth factor-beta superfamily that is secreted by erythroid precursors and other tissues. It has been identified as an oxygen-regulated transcript responding to hypoxia and as a molecule involved in hepcidin regulation. It was suggested that GDF15 overexpression arising from an expanded erythroid compartment contributed to iron overload in thalassemia syndromes by inhibiting hepcidin expression, possibly by antagonizing the BMP pathway [89,93]. GDF15 mRNA levels and secreted protein were up-regulated in response to iron depletion in a range of human cell lines and "in vivo" in humans and this up-regulation was independent of HIF suggesting the existence of a novel iron and oxygen-sensing pathway [106]. Finally, the observation that GDF15 was induced by over-expression of wild type ferroportin connects the iron-mediated regulation of GDF15 concentration to patho-physiological levels of iron. Despite systemic iron overload, ineffective erythropoiesis and associated iron-fluxes in beta-thalassemia might generate an iron deficiency signal in a relevant molecular or cellular context and consequent stimulation of GDF15 expression in a particular erythroid compartment [106]. Experimental data provided the evidence that TWSG1 could be potentially involved in the regulation of hepcidin by erythropoiesis. In contrast to GDF15, the expression of human twisted gastrulation factor (TWSG1) occurs early during erythroblast maturation before hemoglobinization of the cells. TWSG1 is another highly expressed serum protein in thalassemia suppressing hepcidin transcription by interfering with BMP signaling either directly, by acting on BMP receptors, or indirectly by influencing circulating BMP2 and BMP4 levels. So it was proposed that TWSG1 might act with GDF15 to dysregulate iron homeostasis in β-thalassemia [107]. Results obtained by HuH7 hepatoma cells cocultered with primary human erythroblasts or erythroleukemic UT7 cells presented a 20- to 35-fold increase of hepcidin expression and identified OsM responsible for this increase of hepcidin levels. In contrast to GDF15 and TWSG1, it was showed that OsM could induce hepcidin transcription in human hepatoma cell lines mainly through the JAK/STAT pathways [108–109].

7. New therapeutic approaches to limit iron absorption in β-thalassemia

For its frequency and severity β-thalassemia represents a significant health problem in various areas of the world. Conventional treatment of thalassemia includes transfusion therapy, iron chelation therapy and, in rare cases, splenectomy. Regular blood transfusions in combination with aggressive iron chelation have been remarkably effective in delaying the onset of iron-related organ failure and improving mortality but, in spite of this, many patients continue to be affected by cardiac disease and other clinical complications, e.g. develop endocrine failure and delayed pubertal maturation. To add that this rigorous life-long treatment regime is

http://dx.doi.org/10.5772/61716

onerous and represents an enormous imposition on quality of life. Allogeneic hemopoietic stem cell transplantation is the only approach that may lead to a definitive cure but it is not available to most patients. The understanding of β-thalassemia pathophysiology has involved more than 50 years of biochemical and biological studies leading to the development of alternative therapies to cure or ameliorate the disease. New potential molecular targets for β-thalassemic therapy can be divided into three categories. To the first category belong the primary targets that include all of the molecular defects that lead to a decrease in β-globin synthesis. Hemopoietic stem cell transplantation (HSCT), gene therapy using viral vectors and antisense mRNA are an example of strategies targeting the primary causes of reduced β-globin expression. To the second category belong the secondary targets including modifiers of chain imbalance in β-thalassemia by increasing of γ-globin synthesis. Gene therapy approaches for the induction of HbF synthesis include transduction of lentiviral vectors incorporating γ-globin/β-LCR, or attemps to promote endogenous gamma-globin expression using artificial transcription factors. Pharmacological approaches for the induction of gamma-synthesis include the treatment with erythropoietin (EPO) preparations, or short chain fatty acid derivatives (SCFADs) or chemotherapeutic agents as hydroxycarbamide (HU) and 5-azacytidine. To the third category belong the tertiary targets that are those directed at treating the complications of β-thalassemia such as iron overloading and oxidative cellular damage [23–25,89]. In recent years increasing experimental evidences indicated that there was a potential for therapeutic intervention in β-thalassemia by means of manipulating iron metabolism [110–113]. In mice that completely lack Stat5 activity, it was observed that cell surface levels of TfR1 on erythroid cells were decreased more than 2-fold suggesting a link between EpoR/Jak/Stat signaling and iron metabolism [114]. Another study suggested a direct involvement of Epo in hepcidin regulation through the transcriptional factor C/EBP alpha [115]. It was also observed a link between Jak2 and FPN1: Jak2 phosphorylates FPN1 following its binding to hepcidin triggering its internalization and degradation [116]. Therefore, Jack2 might represent one of the major links at the interface between erythropoiesis and iron metabolism suggesting that use of Jak2 inhibitors, antioxidant, and analog of the hepcidin might reduce ineffective erythropoiesis and abnormal iron absorption. Several JAK2 inhibitors have already been developed, showing significant and beneficial results in myelofibrosis and JAK2-related polycythemia vera [117]. However, trials with JAK2 inhibitors in myeloproliferative disorders have also shown several side effects, among them thrombocytopenia and anemia. On the contrary, in preclinical thalassemic models, splenomegaly was reversed in less than two weeks and no side effects were observed [117]. Administration of synthetic hepcidin or of agents that increase its expression, may be beneficial in controlling absorption of this metal. Hepcidin agonists or stimulators of hepcidin production are being developed for the treatment or prevention of iron overload in hepcidin deficiency states, including hereditary hemochromatosis and β-thalassemia. It was observed that transgenic hepcidin therapy improved iron overload as well as erythropoiesis in the mouse model of β-thalassemia [118]. The rationale for the use of hepcidin agonists is justified by two principal observations: first, the phlebotomy is an inexpensive and effective treatment for iron overload that is acceptable to must but not all patients affected by hereditary hemochromatosis; second, the iron-loading anemias cannot be treated in this manner and require iron chelation therapy, which is not well tolerated by many patients. Hepcidin agonists are agents that replace hepcidin activity or stimulate its endogenous production and, in both of hereditary hemochromatosis and iron-loading anemias, could prevent iron accumulation by redistributing iron from parenchymal tissues to macrophages where iron is less toxic. Results obtained treating a mouse model of β-thalassemia with hepcidin agonists suggested that the use of these agents could not only prevent iron overload but could also improve erythropoiesis, perhaps by decreasing excessive alpha-globin synthesis or diminishing oxidative stress in erythropoietic precursors [119–120]. Minihepcidins are short peptide mimetics (9AA long) that are sufficient to induce FPN1 degradation in reporter cells. The extracellular loop of ferroportin surrounding the thiol cysteine C326 appears to be essential for hepcidin binding, as indicated by the lack of hepcidin binding to otherwise fully functional ferroportin containing the isosteric mutation C3265 [119]. Analysis of the interface between hepcidin and ferroportin showed that the segment composed of a 9 N-terminal amino acid segment of hepcidin is sufficient for binding and internalization of ferroportin [121]. These small modified mini-hepcidin peptides show bioactivity in vivo, as determined by their ability to induce hypoferremia in mice and to prevent iron accumulation in hepcidin-deficient mice [119]. Potential drug target also is the transmembrane protease serine 6 (TMPRSS6) or Matriptase-2, a transmembrane serine protease that attenuates hepcidin expression. The fundamental role of TMPRSS6 on hepcidin expression is underscored by the observation that patients and mice with mutations in this gene are affected by iron-refractory iron deficiency anemia (IRIDA) [117]. In Hbbth3/+ mice, use of both antisens oligonucleotide (Tmprss6-ASO9) and RNA interference (Tmprss6-siRNA) can reduce the synthesis of transmembrane serine protease TMPRSS6 by degrading the corresponding mRNA. This led to increased hepcidin expression, decreased Tf-sat, and reduction of hemichrome formation and apoptosis in erythroid cells suggesting that these Tmprss6 inhibitors could be beneficial in individuals with β-thalassemia [117]. Hepcidin levels can be also altered by targeting a bone morphogenetic protein-dependent (BMP-dependent) pathway known to be central to the regulation of hepcidin expression. This pathway involves a multitude of extracellular factors such as GDF15 and TWSG1. These factors are both BMP antagonists produced by erythroblasts that inhibit hepcidin expression in vitro, suggesting their role as putative components of the erythroid regulator [122]. A major goal of hemoglobinopathy research is to develop treatments that correct the underlying molecular defects responsible for β-thalassemia. One approach to achieving this goal is the reactivation of γ-globin synthesis by farmacologic induction. Many of the events controlling the activity of the β-globin locus are known, but the details of those regulating normal human hemoglobin switching and reactivation of HbF in adult hematopoietic cells remain to be elucidated. Agents that increase human HbF in patients may work at one or more levels: for example, hydroxyurea and 5-azacytidine kill dividing cells preferentially and may increase γ-globin expression indirectly through this effect; butyrate may work both by increasing γ-globin translation on ribosomes and by inhibition of histone deacetylase (HDAC) [39, 112,123]. It was showed that Stem Cell Factor (SCF) induced an "in vitro" expansion of effective erythropoiesis and a reactivation of γ-globin synthesis up to fetal levels, paving the way to its potential use in the therapeutic treatment of this disease [124]. Recently it was reported the ability of thalidomide to increase γ-globin gene expression and the proportion of HbF-containing cells in a human "in vitro" erythroid differentiation system. This study has also showed that thalidomide induced production of ROS causing p38 MAPF phosphorylation and globally increased histone H4 acetylation [125]. However, the mecha-

http://dx.doi.org/10.5772/61716

nisms of action of these agents are not yet defined and their role in β-thalassemia therapy is still being explored in light of its acceptable toxicity profiles adding to their promise as therapeutic agents. Key genes controlling fetal/adult globin switching have been identified (e.g. BCL11 and cMYB) and may ultimately serve as direct targets for small molecules that would increase HbF levels in β-thalassemic patients [126–127]. Finally, the fact that most HbF-inducing agents are cytotoxic and many activate the p38MAPK cell stress signaling pathway suggested the importance of what has been termed the "integrated stress response" pathway in erythroid cells to understanding HbF induction. A variety of stress stimuli activate this pathway in erythroid cells: viral infection, ROS, heat shock, NO, ultraviolet irradiation, endoplasmic reticulum stress, inadequate nutrients, proteasome inhibition and limiting amounts of heme [112].

8. Conclusion

The discovery of hepcidin and its role in iron homeostasis has revolutionized our understanding of the pathogenesis of iron overload and iron-restricted anemias and has stimulated the development of new diagnostic and therapeutic methods for these disorders. Several physiological stimuli regulate the production of the iron-regulatory hormone hepcidin: iron loading, inflammation, and erythropoiesis. These stimuli modulate iron availability for erythropoiesis and other physiological processes and regulate the level of body iron stores by altering hepcidin levels. However, important scientific questions still remain to be answered. Further work is required to understand the mechanisms of hepcidin regulation by iron and erythroid activity; to elucidate the structure, the transport function and the complex regulation of the hepcidin receptor ferroportin; to define the hepcidin role in iron homeostasis. In the coming years, these efforts are likely to yield new therapeutical approaches for the treatment of anemia and iron overload disorders.

Acknowledgements

I thank Andrea Occhetti for his contribution to the figures and tables.

Author details

Nadia Maria Sposi*

Address all correspondence to: nadia.sposi@iss.it

Department of Hematology, Oncology and Molecular Medicine, Istituto Superiore di Sanità, Rome, Italy

References

[1] Galanello R, Origa R. Beta-thalassemia. Orphanet J Rare Dis. 2010;21:5–11. DOI: 10.1186/1750–1172–5–11.

[2] Flint J, Harding RM, Boyce AJ, Clegg JB. The population genetics of the hemoglobinopathies. Baillieres Clin Haematol. 1998;11(1):1–51.

[3] Weatherall DJ, Clegg JB, Higgs DR and Wood WG. The hemoglobinopathies. In: Scriver CR, Beaudet AL, Sly WS, Valle D, Vogelstein B, editors. The Metabolic and Molecular Bases of Inherited Disease (OMMBID); Chapter 101. New York, NY: McGraw-Hill. 2002.

[4] Cao A, Galanello R. Beta-thalassemia Genet Med. 2010;12(2):61–76.

[5] Wood B, Higgs D. Molecular basis of thalassemia syndromes. ESH Handbook on Disorders of Erythropoiesis, Erythrocytes and Iron Metabolism. 2009;chapter 10:250–263.

[6] Galanello R, Cao A. Relationship between genotype and phenotype. Thalassemia intermedia. Ann NY Acad Sci. 1998;850:325–333.

[7] Weatherall D. The molecular basis for phenotypic variability of the common thalassemias. Mol Med Today. 1995;1:15–20.

[8] Camaschella C, Mazza U, Roetto A, Gottardi E, Parziale A, Travi M, Fattore S, Bacchiega D, Fiorelli G, Cappellini MD. Genetic interactions in thalassemia intermedia: Analysis of beta-mutations, alpha-genotype, gamma-promoters, and beta-LCR hypersensitive sites 2 and 4 in Italian patients. Am J Hematol. 1995;48(2):82–87.

[9] Cappellini MD, Musallam KM, Cesaretti C, Taher A. Thalassemia intermedia. ESH Handbook on Disorders of Herythropoiesis, Erythrocytes and Iron Metabolism. 2009;chapter 12:286–309.

[10] Li Q, Peterson KR, Fang X, Stamatoyannopoulos G. Locus control regions. Blood. 2002;100:3077–3086.

[11] Palstra RJ, de Laat W, Grosveld F. β-globin regulation and long-rage interactions. Adv Genet. 2008;61:107–142.

[12] Higgs DR, Engel JD, Stamatoyannopoulos G.Thalassemia. Lancet. 2012;379:373–383.

[13] Schrier SL. Pathophysiology of thalassemia. Curr Opin Hematol. 2002;9(2):123–126.

[14] Nienhuis AW, Nathan DG. Pathophysiology and clinical manifestations of the β-thalassemias. Cold Spring Harb Perspect Med. 2012 Dec. 1;2(12):a011726.

[15] Boyer SH, Belding TK, Margolet L, Noyes AN. Fetal hemoglobin restriction to a few erythrocytes (F cells) in normal human adults. Science. 1975;188:361–363.

[16] Uda M, Galanello R, Sanna S, Lettre G, Sankaran VG, Chen W, Usala G, Busonero F, Maschio A, Albai G, Piras MG, Sestu N, Lai S, Dei M, Mulas A, Crisponi L, Naitza S, Asunis I, Deiana M, Nagaraja R, Perseu L, Satta S, Cipollina MD, Sollaino C, Moi P, Hirschhorn JN, Orkin SH, Abecasis GR, Schlessinger D, Cao A. Genome-wide association study shows BCL11A associated with persistent fetal hemoglobin and amelioration of the phenotype of beta-thalassemia. Proc Natl Acad Sci U S A. 2008;105(5): 1620–1625.

[17] Aessopos A, Farmakis D, Deftereos S, Tsironi M, Tassiopoulos S, Moyssakis I, Karagiorga M. Thalassemia heart disease: A comparative evaluation of thalassemia major and thalassemia intermedia. Chest. 2005;127(5):1523–1530.

[18] Telfer P, Coen PG, Christou S, Hadjigavriel M, Kolnakou A, Pangalou E, Pavlides N, Psiloines M, Simamonian K, Skordos G, Sitarou M, Angastiniotis M. Survival of medically treated thalassemia patients in Cyprus. Trends and risk factors over the period 1980-2004. Haematologica. 2006;91(9):1187–1192.

[19] Modell B, Khan M, Darlison M, Westwood MA, Ingram D, Pennell DJ. Improved survival of thalassaemia major in the UK and relation to T2* cardiovascular magnetic resonance. J Cardiovasc Magn Reson. 2008;10:42.

[20] Stamatoyannopoulos G, Grosveld F. Hemoglobin switching. In: Stamatoyannopoulos G, Majerus PW, Pelmutter RM, Vermus H, editors. The molecular basis of blood diseases. 3rd edn. Philadelphia: WB Saunders Company. 2001;136:82.

[21] Weatherall DJ, Clegg JB. The thalassemia syndrome, 4th edn. Oxford: Blackwell Science, 2001.

[22] Voon HP, Vadolas J. Controlling α-globin: A review of α-globin expression and its impact on β-thalassemia. Haematologica. 2008;93:1868–1876.

[23] Thein SL. Genetic modifiers of the β-haemoglobinopathies. Br J Haematol. 2008;141:357–366.

[24] Pace BS, Zein S. Understanding mechanisms of γ-globin gene regulation to develop strategies for pharmacological fetal hemoglobin induction. Dev Dyn. 2006;235:1727–1737.

[25] Perrine SP. Fetal globin stimulant therapies in the β-hemoglobinopathies: Principle and current potential. Pediatr Ann. 2008;37:339–346.

[26] Trompeter S, Roberts I. Hemoglobin F modulation in childhood sickle cell disease. Br J Hematol. 2009;144:308–316.

[27] Orkin SH, Zon LI. Hematopoiesis: an evolving paradigm for stem cell biology. Cell. 2008;132(4):631–644.

[28] Palis J. Ontogeny of erythropoiesis. Current Opinion in Hematology. 2008;15(3):155–161.

[29] Tsiftsoglou AS, Vizirianakis IS, Strouboulis J. Erythropoiesis: Model systems, molecular regulators, and developmental programs. IUBMB Life. 2009;61(8):800–830.

[30] Weissman IL. Stem cells: Units of development, units of regeneration, and units in evolution. Cell. 2000;100(1):157–168.

[31] Ingley E, Tilbrook PA, Klinken SP. New insights into the regulation of erythroid cells. IUMBMB Life. 2004;56(4):177–184.

[32] Koury MJ, Sawyer ST, Brandt SJ. New insights into erythropoiesis. Current Opinion in Hematology. 2002;9(2):93–100.

[33] Stamatoyannopoulos G. Control of globin gene expression during development and erythroid differentiation. Experimental Hematology. 2005;33(3):259–271.

[34] Cianetti L, Gabbianelli M, Sposi NM. Ferroportin and erythroid cells: An update. Advance in Hematology. 2010; vol. 2010, Article ID 404173, 12 pages.

[35] Golde DW. The stem cell. Scientific American. 1991;265(6):86–93.

[36] Metcalf D. The molecular control of cell division, differentiation committment and maturation in hemopoietic cells. Nature. 1989;339(6219):27–30.

[37] Orkin SH. Development of the hematopoietic system. Current Opinion in Genetics and Development. 1996;6(5):597–602.

[38] Emerson SG, Thomas S, Ferrara JL, Greenstein JL. Developmental regulation of erythropoiesis by hematopoietic growth factors: Analysis on populations of BFU-E from bone marrow, peripheral blood, and fetal liver. Blood. 1989;74(1):49–55.

[39] Sposi NM. Relationship between iron and erythropoiesis. In: Sarika Arora (Ed) Iron Metabolism. ISBN: 978–953–51–0605–0. InTech. 2011;61–86.

[40] Domen J, Weissman IL. Self-renewal, differentiation or death: Regulation and manipulation of hematopoietic stem cell fate. Molecular Medicine Today. 1999;5(5):201–208.

[41] Ogawa M. Differentiation and proliferation of hematopoietic stem cells. Blood. 1993;81(11):2844–2853.

[42] Grover CB Jr. Hematopoiesis. The molecular basic of blood. 1994, Sander ed.

[43] Bernstein ID, Andrews RG, Zsebo KM. Recombinant human stem cell factor enhances the formation of colonies by CD34+ and CD34 + lin- cells, and the generation of colony-forming cell progeny from CD34 + lin- cells cultured with interleukin-3, granulocyte colony-stimulating factor, or granulocyte-macrofage colony-stimulating factor. Blood 1991;77(11):2316–2321.

[44] Gabbianelli M, Pelosi E, Montesoro E, Valtieri M, Luchetti L, Samoggia P, Vitelli L, Barbieri T, Testa U, Peschle C. Multi-level effects of flt3 ligand on human hematopoiesis: Expansion of putative stem cells and proliferation of granulomonocytic progenitors/monocytic precursors. Blood 1995;86(5):1661–1670.

[45] Lyman SD, James L, Johnson L, Brasel K, De Vries P, Escobar SS, Downwy H, Splett RR, Beckmann MP, McKenna HJ. Cloning of the human homolog of the murine flt3 ligand: A growth factor for early hematopoietic progenitor cells. Blood. 1994;83(10): 2795–2801.

[46] Berardi AC, Wang A, Abraham J, Scadden DT. Basic fibroblast growth factor mediates its effects on committed myeloid progenitors by direct action and has no effect on hematopoietic stem cells. Blood. 1995;86(6):2123–2129.

[47] Gabbianelli M, Sargiacomo M, Pelosi E, Testa U, Isacchi G, Peschle C. Pure human hematopoietic progenitors: Permissive action of basic fibroblast growth factor. Science. 1990;249(4976):1561–1564.

[48] Leary AG, Ikebuchi K, Hirai Y, Wong GG, Yang YC, Clark SC, ad Ogawa M. Sinergism between interlukin-6 and interleukin-3 in supporting proliferation of human hematopoietic stem cells: comparison with interleukin-1 alpha. Blood. 1988;71(6): 1759–1763.

[49] Metcalf D. Hematopoietic regulators: Redundancy or subtlety? Blood. 1993;82(12): 3515–3523.

[50] Fried W. Erythropoietin. Annual Review of Nutrition. 1995;15:353–377.

[51] Krantz SB. Erythropoietin. Blood. 1991;77(3):419–434.

[52] Demetri GD, Griffin JD. Granulocyte colony-stimulating factor and its receptor. Blood. 1991; 78(11):2791–2808.

[53] Sherr CJ. Colony-stimulatin factor-1 receptor. Blood. 1990;75(1):1–12.

[54] Kaushanky K, Lok S, Holly RD, Broudy VC, Lin N, Bailey MC, Forstrom JW, Buddle MM, Oort PJ, Hagen FS, Roth GJ, Papayannopoulou T, Foster DC. Promotion of megakaryocyte progenitor expansion and differentiation by the c-Mpl ligand thrombopoietin. Nature. 1994;369(6481):568–571.

[55] Testa U, Pelosi E, Peschle C. The transferrin receptor. Critical Reviews in Oncogenesis. 1993;4(3):241–276.

[56] Testa U. Recent developments in the understanding of iron metobolism. The Hematology Journal. 2002;3(2)63–89.

[57] Loken MR, Shah VO, Dattilio KL, Civin CI. Flow cytometric analysis of human bone marrow: I. Normal erythroid development. Blood. 1987;69(1):255–263.

[58] Okumura N, Tsuji K, Nakahata T. Changes in cell surface antigen expressions during proliferation and differentiation of human erythroid progenitors. Blood. 1992;80(3): 642–650.

[59] Ponka P. Tissue-specific regulation of iron metabolism and heme synthesis: Distinct control mechanisms in erythorid cells. Blood. 1997;89(1):1–25.

[60] Andrews NC. Iron homeostasis: Insights from genetics and animal models. Nature Reviews. Genetics. 2000;1(3):208–217.

[61] Gregory T, Yu C, Ma A, Orkin H, Blobel GA, Weiss Mj. GATA-1 and erythropoietin cooperate to promote erythroid cell survival by regulating bcl-x(L) expression. Blood. 1999;94(1): 87–96.

[62] Kim SI, Bresnik EH. Transcriptional control of erythropoiesis: Emerging mechanisms and principles. Oncogene. 2007;26:6777–6794.

[63] Ribeil JA, Arlet JB, Dussiot M, Moura IC, Courtois G, Hermine O. Ineffective erythropoiesis in β-thalassemia. Hindawi Publishing Corporation. The Scientific World Journal. 2013;2013, Article ID 394295, 11 pages.

[64] Fang J, Menon M, Kapelle W, Bogacheva O, Bogachev O, Houde E, Browne S, Sathyanarayana P, Wojchowski DM. Epo modulation of cell-cycle regulatory genes, and cell division, in primary bone marrow erythroblasts. Blood. 2007;110:2361–2370.

[65] Socolovsky M, Murrel M, Liu Y, Pop R, Porpiglia E, Levchenko A. Negative autoregolation by FAS mediates robust fetal erythropoiesis. PLoS Biology. 2007;5(10):article e252.

[66] Menon MP, Karuz V, Bogachava O, Bogachev O, Cuetara B, Wojchowski DM. Signals for stress erythropoiesis are integrated via an erythropoietin receptor-phosphotyrosine 343-Stat5 axis. Journal of Clinical Investigation. 2006;116:683–694.

[67] Hengartner MO. The biochemistry of apoptosis. Nature. 2000;407:770–776.

[68] Yi CH, Yuan J. The Jekyll and hyde functions of caspases. Developmental Cell. 2009;16(1):21–34.

[69] Visvader JE, Mao X, Fujiwara Y, Hahm K, Orkin SH. The LIM-domain binding protein Ldb1 and its partner LMO2 act as negative regulators of erythroid differentiation. Proc Natl Acad Sci USA. 1997;94(25):13,707–13,712.

[70] Beaumont C, Vaulont S. Iron homeostasis. ESH Handbook Disorders of iron homeostasis, erythrocytes, erythropoiesis. 2006;Cap.18:393–406.

[71] Hentze MW, Muckenthaler MV, Andrews NC. Balancing acts: Molecular control of mammalian iron metabolism. Cell. 2004;117:285–297.

[72] Yun S, Vincelette ND. Update on iron metabolism and molecular perspective of common genetic and acquired disorder, hemochromatosis. Crit Rev. Oncol Hematol. 2015 Feb. 18. pii: S1040-8428(15)00,030-X. doi: 10.1016/j.critrevonc.2015.02.006.

[73] Munoz M, Villar I, Garcia-Erce JA. An update on iron physiology. World J Gastroenterol. 2009;15(37):4617–4626.

[74] Andrews NC. Disorders of iron metabolism. N Engl J Med. 1999;341:1986–1995.

[75] Siah CW, Ombiga J, Adams LA, Trinder D, Olynyc JK. Normal iron metabolism and the pathophysiology of iron overload disorders. Clin Biochem Rev. 2006;27:5–16.

[76] Fleming RE, Bacon BR. Orchestration of iron homeostasis. N Engl J Med. 2005;352:1741–1744.

[77] Coates TD. Physiology and pathophysiology of iron in hemoglobin-associated diseases. Free Radical Biology and medicine 2014;72:23–40.

[78] Anderson CP, Shen M, Eisenstein RS, Leibold EA. Mammalian iron metabolism and its control by iron regulatory proteins. Biochim. Biophys. Acta. 2012;1823:1468–1483.

[79] Hubert N, Hentze MW. Previously uncharacterized isoforms of divalent metal transporter (DMT)-1: Implications for regulation and cellular function. Proc Natl Acad Sci USA. 2002;99:12,345–12,350.

[80] Anderson GJ, Frazer DM, Mc Laren GD. Iron absorption and metabolism. Curr Opin Gastroenterol. 2009;25:129–135.

[81] Donovan A, Roy CN, Andrews NC. The ins and outs of iron homeostasis. Physiology (Bethesda). 2006;21:115–123.

[82] Evstatiev R, Gasche C. Iron sensing and signaling. Gut. 2012;61:933–952.

[83] Fleming RE, Ponka P. Iron overload in human disease. N Engl J Med. 2012;366:348:359.

[84] Park CH, Valore EV, Waring AJ, Ganz T. Hepcidin, a urinary antimicrobial peptide synthesized in the liver. Journal of Biological Chemistry. 2001;276:7806–7810.

[85] Nicolas G, Bennoun M, Devaux I, Beaumont C, Grandchamp B, Kahn A, Vaulont S. Lack of hepcidin gene expression and severe tissue iron overload in upstream stimulatory factor 2 (USF2) knockout mice. Proc Natl Acad Sci USA. 2001;98:8780–8785.

[86] Fleming RE, Sly WS. Hepcidin: A putative iron regulatory hormone relevant to hereditary hemochromatosis and the anemia of chronic disease. Proc Natl Acad Sci USA. 2001;98:8160–8162.

[87] Nicolas G, Chauvet C, Viatte L, Danan JL, Bigard X, Devaux I, Beaumont C, Kahn A, Vaulont S. The gene encoding the iron regulatory peptide hepcidin is regulated by anemia, hypoxia and inflammation. Journal of Clinical Investigation. 2002;110:1037–1044.

[88] Ganz T. Cellular iron: Ferroportin is the only way out. Cell Metabolism. 2005;1:155–157.

[89] Piperno A, Mariani R, Trombini P, Girelli D. Hepcidin modulation in human diseases: From research to clinic. World Journal of Gastroenterology. 2009;15:538–551.

[90] Andrews NC. Forging a field: The golden age of iron biology. Blood. 2008;112:219–230.

[91] Rivella S. The role of ineffective erythropoiesis in non-transfusion dependent thalassemia. Blood Rev. 2012;26(Suppl.1):512–515.

[92] Pasricha SR, Frazer DM, Bowden DK, Anderson GJ. Transfusion suppresses erythropoiesis and increases hepcidin in adult patients with beta-thalassemia major: A longitudinal study. Blood. 2013;122:124–133.

[93] Tanno T, Bhanu NV, Oneal PA, Goh SH, Staker P, Lee YT, Moroney JW, Reed CH, Luban NL, Wang RH, Eling TE, Childs R, Ganz T, Leitman SF, Fucharoen S, Miller JL. High levels of GDF15 in thalassemia suppress expression of the iron regulatory protein hepcidin. Nat Med. 2007;13:1096–1101.

[94] Silvestri L, Pagani A, Camaschella C. Furin-mediated release of soluble hemojuvelin: A new link between hypoxia and iron homeostasis. Blood. 2008;111:924–931.

[95] Kautz L, Jung G, Nemeth E, Ganz T. The erythroid factor erythroferrone and its role in iron homeostasis. Blood. 2013;122 (21).

[96] Kautz L, Jung G, Valore EV, Rivella S, Nemeth E, Ganz T. Identification of erythroferrone as an erythroid regulator of iron metabolism. Nature Genet. 2014;46:678–684.

[97] Kautz L, Nemeth E. Molecular liaisons between erythropoiesis and iron metabolism. Blood. 2014;124:479–482.

[98] Melchiori L, Gardenghi S, Rivella S. β-thalassemia: HiJAKing ineffective erythropoiesis and iron overload. Adv Haematol. 2010;2010:938,640.

[99] Pippard MS, Callender ST, Warner GT, Weatherall DJ. Iron absorption and loading in β-thalassemia intermedia. The Lancet. 1979;8147:819–821.

[100] Gardenghi S, Marongiu MF, Ramos P, Guy E, Breda L, Chadburn A, Liu Y, Amariglio N, Rechavi G, Rachmilewitz EA, Brener W, Cabantchik ZI, Wrighting DM, Andrews NC, de Sousa M, Giardina PJ, Grady RW, Rivella S. Ineffective erythropoiesis in beta-thalassemia is characterized by increased iron absorption mediated by down-regulation of hepcidin and up-regulation of ferroportin. Blood. 2007;109:5027–5035.

[101] Rivella S. Ineffective erythropoiesis and thalassemias. Current Opinion in Hematology. 2009;16:187:194.

[102] Ganz T. Hepcidin, a key regulator of iron metabolism and mediator of anemia of inflammation. Blood. 2003;102:783–788.

[103] Papanikolaou G, Tzilianos JI, Christakis JI, Bogdanos D, Tsimirika K, MacFarlane J, Goldberg YP, Sakellaropoulos N, Ganz T, Nemeth E. Hepcidin in iron overload disorders. Blood. 2005;105:4103–4105.

[104] Kattamis A, Papassotiriou I, Palaiologou D, Apostolakou F, Galani A, Ladis V, Sakellaropoulos N, Papanikolaou G. The effects of erythropoietic activity and iron burden on hepcidin expression in patients with thalassemia major. Haematologica. 2006;91:809–812.

[105] Weizer-Stern O, Adamsky K, Amariglio N, Levin C, Koren A, Breuer W, Rachmilewitz E, Breda L, Rivella S, Cabantchik ZI, Rechavi G. Downregulation of hepcidin and haemojuvelin expression in the hepatocyte cell-line HepG2 induced by thalassemic sera. British Journal of Hematology. 2006;135:129–138.

[106] Lakhal S, Talbot NP, Crosby A, Stoepker C, Townsend AR, Robbins PA, Pugh CW, Ratcliffe PJ, Mole DR. Regulation of growth differentiation factor 15 expression by intracellular iron. Blood. 2009;113:1555–1563.

[107] Tanno T, Porayette P, Sripichai O, Noh SJ, Byrnes C, Bhupatiraju A, Lee YT, Goodnough JB, Harandi O, Ganz T, Paulson RF, Miller JL. Identification of TWSG1 as a second novel erythroid regulator of hepcidin expression in murin and human cells. Blood. 2009;114:181–186.

[108] Chung B, Verdier F, Matak P, Deschemin JC, Mayeux P, Vaulont S. Oncostatin M is a potent inducer of hepcidin, the iron regulatory hormone. The FASEB Journal. 2010;24:2093–2103.

[109] Kanda J, Uchiyama T, Tomosugi N, Higuchi M, Uchiyama T, Kawabata H. Oncostatin M and leukemia inhibitory factor increase hepcidin expression in hepatoma cell lines. International Journal of Hematology. 2009;90:545–552.

[110] Nemeth E. Iron regulation and erythropoiesis. Curr Opin Hematol. 2008;15:169–175.

[111] Tsiftsoglou AS, Tsamadou AI, Papadopoulou LC. Heme as key regulator of major mammalian cellular functions: molecular, cellular and pharmacological aspects. Pharmacology and Therapeutics. 2006;11:327–345.

[112] Mabaera R, West RJ, Conine SJ, Macari ER, Boyd CD, Engman CA, Lowrey CH. A cell stress signaling model of fetal hemoglobin induction: What doesn't kill red blood cells may make them stronger. Experimental Hematology. 2008;36:1057–1072.

[113] Rund D, Rachmilewitz E. Beta-thalassemia. New England Journal of Medicine. 2005;353:1135–1146.

[114] Kerenyi MA, Grebien F, Gehart H, Schifrer M, Artaker M, Kovacic B, Beug H, Moriggi R, Mullner EW. Stat5 regulates cellular iron uptake of erythroid cells via IRP-2 and TfR1. Blood. 2008;112:3878–3888.

[115] Pinto JP, Ribeiro S, Pontes H, Thowfeequ S, Tosh D, Carvalho F, Porto G. Erythropoietin mediates hepcidin expression in hepatocytes through EPOR signaling and regulation of C/EBP (alpha). Blood. 2008;111:5727–5733.

[116] De Domenico I, Lo E, Ward DM, Kaplan J. Hepcidin-induced internalization of ferroportin requires binding and cooperative interaction with Jak2. Proceedings of the National Academy of Sciences of the United States of America. 2009;106:3800–3805.

[117] Rivella S. β-thalassemias: Paradigmatic diseases for scientific discoveries and development of innovative therapies. Haematologica. 2015;100(4):418–430.

[118] Ganz T. Hepcidin and iron regulation, 10 years later. Blood. 2011;117:4425–4433.

[119] Ganz T, Nemeth E. The hepcidin-ferroportin system as a therapeutic target in anemias and iron overload. Hematology Am Soc Hematol Educ Program. 2011;2011:538–542.

[120] Gardenghi S, Ramos P, Marongiu MF, Melchiori L, Breda L, Guy E, Muirhead K, Rao N, Roy CN, Andrews NC, Nemeth E, Follenzi A, An X, Mohandas N, Ginzburg Y, Rachmilewitz EA, Giardina PJ, Grady RW, Rivella S. Hepcidin as a therapeutic tool to limit iron overload and improve anemia in β-thalassemic mice. J Clin Invest. 2010;120:4466–4477.

[121] Preza GC, Ruchala P, Pinon R, Ramos E, Quiao B, Peralta MA, Sharma S, waring A, Ganz T, Nemeth E. Minihepcidin are rationally designed small peptides that mimic hepcidin activity in mice and may be useful for the treatment of iron overload. J Clin Invest. 2011;121:4880–4888.

[122] Bartnikas TB, Fleming MD. A tincture of hepcidin cures all: The potential for hepcidin therapeutics. J Clin Invest. 2010;120:4187–4190.

[123] Bank A. Regulation of human fetal hemoglobin: New player, new complexities. Blood. 2006;107:435–443.

[124] Gabbianelli M, Morsilli O, Massa A, Pasquini L, Cianciulli P, Testa U, Peschle C. Effective erythropoiesis and HbF reactivation induced by kit ligand in beta-thalassemia. Blood. 2008;11:421–429.

[125] Aerbajinai W, Zhu J, Gao Z, Chin K, Rodgers GP. Thalidomide induces gamma-globin gene expression through increased reactive oxygen species-mediated p38 MAPK signaling and histone H4 acetylation in adult erythropoiesis. Blood. 2007;110:2864–2871.

[126] Ginzburg Y, Rivella S. β-thalassemia: A model for elucidating the dynamic regulation of ineffective erythropoiesis and iron metabolism. Blood. 2011;118:4321–4330.

[127] Wilber A, Nienhuis AW, Persons DA. Transcriptional regulation of fetal to adult hemoglobin switching: A new therapeutic opportunities. Blood. 2011;117: 3945–3953.

Chapter 5

Acute Splenic Sequestration Crisis

Jorge Peña Siado and Julian Londono Hernández

Additional information is available at the end of the chapter

http://dx.doi.org/10.5772/60811

Abstract

Acute splenic sequestration crisis (ASSC) is a life-threatening complication associated with sickle cell anemia (SCA) that consists of an acute fall in hemoglobin produced by red blood cell (RBC) sickling within the spleen. It is also one of the leading causes of death in children with SCA. Occlusion of the splenic vascular supply leads to parenchymal ischemia and tissue necrosis. ASSCs are considered an emergency because of their high morbidity and mortality. Untreated patients may die within 1–2 h due to circulatory failure. Management is supportive, sometimes with blood transfusion and total or partial splenectomy.

The aim of this chapter is to bring the up-to-date knowledge of the epidemiology, pathophysiology, diagnosis, and treatment of ASCC. Other important items considered are the spleen dysfunction, susceptibility to infections, and its prevention, disease expression, and to address the different managements for improving prognosis.

Keywords: Sickle cell anemia (SCA), acute splenic sequestration crisis (ASSC), splenomegaly, hypersplenism, splenectomy

1. Introduction

In 1904, Herrick was the first to describe sickle cell anemia (SCA) in a West Indian student [1]. SCA is one of the most frequent hemoglobinopathies in the world. This disease may affect any part of the body, and one of the most commonly affected organs is the spleen. This disease results from a change of the amino acid valine instead of glutamic acid in the sixth position of the beta chain of hemoglobin. This change will produce rigid sickle-shaped red blood cells (RBCs) that hemolyze easily and adhere to each other blocking blood vessels [2].

The SCA is associated with several problems that can acutely or chronically affect health of children or adults with this disease: vasoocclusive crisis, aplastic crisis, acute splenic crisis sequestration, acute chest syndrome, stroke, priapism, and impaired growth and development. This type of anemia is inherited in an autosomal recessive manner. When there is only one abnormal copy of the gene, patients do not experience symptoms [3].

In children with SCA, spleen may be clinically palpable or not, functional or not, and not have existing correlation between size and function. The spleen is the organ most affected in SCA. Often, hyposplenism occurs before 1 year of age. Autosplenectomy is caused by fibrosis of the spleen as a result of multiple repeated vasoocclusive crises and usually is present between 5 and 6 years. Splenomegaly, sometimes with hypersplenism, can occur with the loss of function of the spleen. Hyposplenism increases the risk of infections with encapsulated bacteria [4].

The first person who conceptualized the term acute splenic sequestration crisis (ASSC) was Topley in 1981, who defined it as acute splenic enlargement with a fall in the hemoglobin (Hb) level of at least 20 g/l (or 2 g/dL) and abnormal basal reticulocyte count [5]. It is also defined as the sudden onset of splenomegaly (greater than 2 cm from the steady-state level) or sudden enlargement of a preexisting splenomegaly in association with acute anemia, evidence of active bone marrow, and regression of splenomegaly after blood transfusion. It is the result of rapid sequestration of RBCs in the spleen, which alters its functioning. ASSC is divided into major and minor [6, 7, 8].Minor ASSC refers to the moderate increase in splenic size and the decrease in Hb level of 2 to 3 g/dL; sometimes reaching a level as low as 2 to 3 g/dL, the spleen size regresses after blood transfusion, and there is evidence of active bone marrow.

Minor ASSC is referred as a moderate increase in splenic size and a decrease in Hb level of 2 to 3 g/dL; the spleen size regresses after blood transfusion, and there is evidence of active bone marrow.

Splenomegaly is the enlargement of the spleen. However, an enlarged or palpable spleen is not necessarily of clinical significance. Moreover, certain individuals with broadly splayed costal margins have readily palpable but small spleens. A spleen weight of 400–500 g indicates splenomegaly, and some authors consider spleens weighing more than 1000 g to have massive splenomegaly. Spleens that are prominent below the costal margin typically weigh 750–1000 g. Poulin et al. defined splenomegaly as moderate if the largest dimension is 11–20 cm and severe if the largest dimension is greater than 20 cm [9].Hypersplenism refers to splenomegaly and any combination of anemia, leucopenia, and thrombocytopenia, with compensatory bone marrow hyperplasia and tendency to normalization of blood parameters after splenectomy [10, 11].Hyposplenism is defined as an acquired disorder caused by several hematological and immunological diseases and characterized by absent or reduced splenic function impairment [12]. The most common condition associated with hyposplenism is sickle cell anemia, but it is also usually due to surgical removal, congenital aplasia, tumor metastasis, splenic vascular accident, alcoholic liver disease, celiac disease, bone marrow transplantation, and inflammatory bowel disease [13]. RBC abnormalities, including the presence of inclusions, nucleated RBC, and target cells, are commonly present. Patients with hyposplenism are at increased risk of bacterial sepsis, especially due to infection by *Streptococcus pneumoniae, Neisseria meningitidis*, and *Haemophilus influenza* type b.Massive splenic infarction (MSI) is the infarction involving more than 50% of the spleen size. MSI is extremely rare in children with SCA. It can develop spontaneously or be precipitated by other factors, namely, high altitude, acute chest syndrome, and severe stress in the form of septicemia or severe vasoocclusive crisis [6, 14].Epidemiology

ASSC is a serious and the earliest life-threatening complication seen in patients with SCA [15]. It may occur during the first weeks of life, and it could be the first symptom of the disease. Up to 75% of first cases occur before 2 years. ASSC is considered the second leading cause of death after infection in the first decade of life in these patients. These crises are usually seen in infants and young children commonly between 5 months and 2 years of age. Mortality is up to 3% in children and 10% of adults who die from hypovolemic shock given the lack of early transfusion. Other reports show mortality rates of 15%–44% [16, 17]. Early neonatal screening and early parental education diminishes mortality rate up to 0.53% [4].Between 10% and 30% of homozygous children have suffered a crisis of splenic sequestration before 3 years of age, and all patients with SCA and no fibrosis spleen are susceptible to ASSC. In homozygous patients, it usually occurs between 3 months and 3 years old, but it can occur at older ages in those treated early with hydroxyurea, delayed autosplenectomy, and also in double heterozygotes SC and S-thalassemia, in which it can occur even in adulthood. There is a recurrence in the 50% of those who survive a first episode of splenic sequestration [11].

In the study of Brousse and colleagues [18], 190 children with SCA diagnosed at birth with SS or Sbeta0 were followed during a study period of 9 years. Among these 190 children are 111 boys and 79 girls (sex ratio, 1:4). They found 437 episodes of ASSC (0.06/patient-year); the median age at the first episode was 1.4 years (0.1–7), and 67% of patients had more than one episode. This study showed that the risk of recurrence was lower when the first episode occurred after 2 years and was higher when the first episode appeared before 1 year of age. In the same study, it was found that patients may experience several episodes, including more than 5; also, the prevalence of ASSC among children with SCA was 12.6%. ASSC incidence was 0.06/patient-year. The lifelong prevalence of acute splenic sequestration ranges from 7% to 30% according to studies [5, 15, 16].Pathophysiology

The spleen is a lymphoid organ dedicated to the clearance of blood cells and pathogens. It links innate and adaptive immune responses. The spleen filters approximately 5% of the cardiac output every minute [19].At present, the pathophysiology of ASSC is not completely understood. In normal conditions, the blood enters to the spleen through the splenic artery and then is distributed through the trabecular arteries that branch throughout the parenchyma to a terminating arteriole called the central arteriole. Splenic arterioles may drain into the venous sinuses or within the parenchyma and thus relieve their blood in the cords of red pulp. The spleen contains specialized macrophages, which are in close contact with blood cells and circulating bacteria, producing phagocytosis of some pathogens [20, 21]. Ten percent of the blood flowing through the spleen passes through filtration beds slowly. There is additional resistance due to the dynamic properties of both endothelial cells, and specialized fibroblasts [22] may play an important role in regulating blood filtration and possibly be dysfunctional in pathological conditions like SCA.The white pulp selectively clears lymphocytes and accessory cells from the blood and allows the spleen to initiate an adaptive immune response. The marginal zone of the spleen produces immunoglobulin M (IgM) that is essential for the phagocytosis of encapsulated bacteria such as *S. pneumoniae* and *H. influenza* type b (Hib). The marginal area is responsible for the generation of IgM by memory B cells. Macrophages in the filtration beds exert functions as erythrophagocytosis and recycling iron [23].The main clinical consequences of defective spleen function derive from the alteration of both the filtering and immune functions, leading to increased susceptibility to bacterial infection, increased risks of vascular complications and autoimmunity [18].

In SCA, RBCs are not deformable enough. The Hb S chain, with valine at the sixth position, has an unusual propensity to bind with other Hb S chains when deoxygenated This polymerization results in rigid molecules of hemoglobin, which are joined to each other and thus it is produced larger polymers that trigger a variety of elongated erythrocytes with decreased deformability. Polymerization in SCA is a process that occurs by factors that lead to deoxygenation such as high altitudes, infections, decreased pH, and low temperatures [24].Polymerization is responsible for the sickled or banana shape of RBCs in SCA, which causes a nonselective increase in membrane cation permeability to sodium, potassium, magnesium, and calcium. When these cations enter the RBC (down their concentration gradient), several cell membrane transport systems are activated, with the important cumulative effect being the egress of water. The polymerization causes erythrocytes with a banana-shaped form that leads to an increase in the permeability of sodium, potassium, magnesium, and calcium. These cations will produce an activation of several transportation systems in the red cell membrane, which leads to dehydration of these cells. When the red cell has had several episodes of polymerization and dehydration, it becomes irreversibly deformed cell, which leads to vasoocclusion [25] (see Figure 1).The normal red blood cell can deform as it passes through small vessels. Dehydrated cells increase their viscosity, leading to a decreased deformability [26].

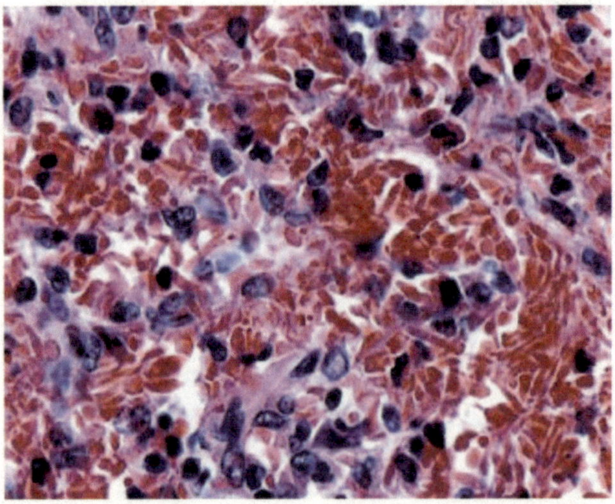

Figure 1. Vascular sinus congestion with Hb SS BCs. Medium-power photomicrograph (original magnification, ×40; hematoxylin–eosin stain) of a spleen tissue sample shows congestion of the vascular sinuses with Hb SS RBCs. (Adopted from Gael J. Sickle cell anemia. RadioGraphics, 2001; 21:971–994.)

2. Etiology

Precipitating factors have been described such as bacterial–viral infections (parvovirus B19) or acute chest syndrome or exposure to high altitudes. Febrile events in SS infants may trigger or promote ASSC [27]. Increased inflammation during a febrile condition or vasoocclusive crisis may promote the trapping of blood within the spleen by increasing blood cellularity, blood viscosity, and erythrocyte rigidity [28]. Other precipitating factors (genetic or environmental) need to be sought in the hope that factors predicting ASSC will eventually be identified. Of note, none of the studied children in some studies had concomitant or secondary acute chest syndrome [16, 29].

3. Diagnosis

As defined previously, the ASSC is a decrease of at least 2 g/dL in Hb concentration from baseline (or fall by 20% hematocrit) and increased reticulocytosis and splenomegaly >2 cm compared to baseline. It can also have thrombocytopenia. The clinical manifestations, laboratory studies, and radiological features may raise the suspect about this condition.

The differentiation of ASSC from similar conditions is imperative. Transient aplastic crisis due to parvovirus B19 infection occurs in older children with SCA and typically manifests as worsening anemia with reticulocytopenia and no splenomegaly [30].Malaria and SCA could be present concomitantly and may exacerbate each other, so it is crucial to rule out coinfections [31].

3.1. Clinical presentation

ASSC manifests clinically as the sudden onset of asthenia, adynamia, pain and abdominal distension, pallor, tachycardia, tachypnea, splenomegaly, thirstiness, decreased activity, decreased oral intake, and increased fussiness, and children could quickly manifest signs and symptoms of hypovolemic shock in severe cases. These crises are transient and usually may last from 3 to 4 h until 1 day. Mallouh et al. [28] found that two-thirds of the patients had a fever or infection at the time of the first ASSC.

The older patients may complain of left-sided abdominal pain. Infants with acute splenic sequestration can have sudden, rapid, massive enlargement of the spleen. The hemoglobin may fall by half of its baseline value within a few hours of onset of the sequestration crisis.

It is important to recognize that the spleen is moderately to markedly enlarged, and sometimes very painful. Diffuse abdominal tenderness may increase the suspect of splenic sequestration.

3.2. Laboratory

All patients should promptly have minimum laboratory studies, such as CBC with differential, reticulocyte, and platelet count, and chemistry profile, including electrolytes, AST, ALT, bilirubin, alkaline phosphatase, LDH, BUN, creatinine, and urinalysis.

As mentioned before thrombocytopenia, leukopenia and elevated reticulocyte count can also be seen in these children and can be useful in the diagnosis. It is necessary to take into account that hepatic sequestration can occur in patients with SCA, and this condition could have a clinical presentation with abdominal pain and hepatomegaly. Findings may include mild to moderate elevation of liver transaminases.

There is no exact functional evaluation of the spleen, but blood markers, such as Howell–Jolly bodies (HJB) or pitted cells (PIT), could assess the filtering function of the spleen [4].

Howell–Jolly bodies are nuclear remnants in circulating mature red cells, which are, in physiological conditions, groomed or pitted by the spleen. The circulating number of HJB can be counted on blood smears or by flow cytometry [32] and has therefore been used as a marker of splenic dysfunction.

3.3. Imaging

Clinical signs make the diagnosis. Imaging is therefore not essential and, if performed, should be planned after treatment has started. Suspicion of splenic abscess in children with SCA, who have fever, abdominal pain, and an enlarged spleen, must be corroborated by ultrasound.

When loss of splenic function is present, the uptake of ^{99m}Tc sulfur colloid diminishes and may entirely disappear. Areas with loss of function could appear as rounded masses of hypoechoic tissue at ultrasound (US) and computed tomography (CT) and may have an attenuation similar to that of normal spleen (see Figure 2A) [33].

The spleen with several ASSC becomes small and calcified. This fibrotic spleen has low signal intensity. These calcifications may be visible at radiography and CT (as shown in Figure 2B).

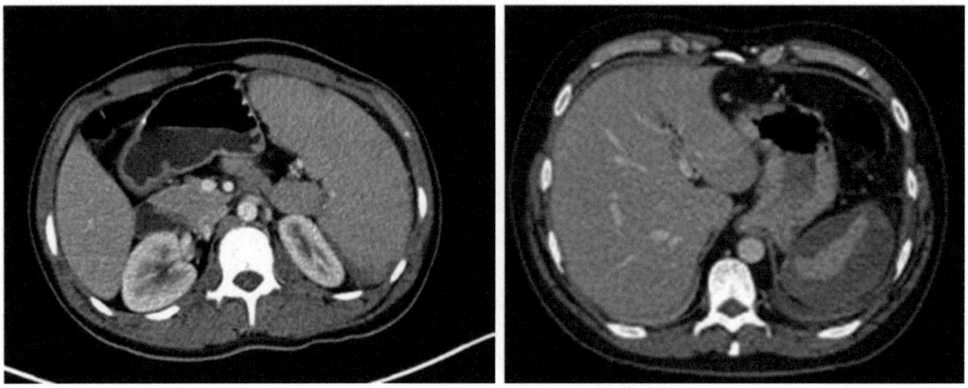

A B

Figure 2. (A) Enlarged spleen with subcapsular infarction in the posterior pole, suggestive of ASSC. (B) Enlarged spleen that enhances heterogeneously with calcifications, suggestive of ASSC in fibrotic phase. (Courtesy of Lina Marcela Cadavid Alvarez, MD, Radiologist.)

http://dx.doi.org/10.5772/60811

4. Treatment

Management is supportive, including the restoration of intravascular volume by packed red blood cell transfusion. The spleen usually decreases its size after a few days or weeks, also resolving thrombocytopenia and leucopenia.

Other support measures include intravenous (IV) fluids such as volume expanders as Ringer lactate or saline solution 0.9%. Transfuse patients with packed RBCs who have acute splenic sequestration and severe anemia to raise the hemoglobin to a stable level. Keep in mind that sequestered red blood cells in the spleen are mobilized after transfusion, so that the level of Hb may increase more than expected.

Do not expect to know the results of additional tests if the suspicion diagnostic request is clear and very urgent transfusion even without cross in case there is evidence of hemodynamic instability. It is recommended to proceed with partial exchange transfusion for signs of respiratory distress [34].

Children younger than 2 years should to ingress in a program of chronic transfusion to maintain HbS <30% until consider splenectomy after that age [35].Discard malaria in patients recently arrived from endemic countries, including PCR by low parasitemia usual [31].

It is important to address the performance and timing of splenectomy in patients with recurrent acute splenic sequestration or symptomatic hypersplenism (see Algorithm 1).

Splenectomy is an essential part of the management of splenic sequestration crisis. Most of the authors recommend splenectomy after the second episode of ASSC. Consider urgent splenectomy if the patient shows no clinical signs of improvement [36]. Splenectomy may be recommended after a first episode if life threatening is predicted.

Within the complications seen after splenectomy are an increased susceptibility to infections by encapsulated bacteria, but other authors have not found an increased incidence of bacteremia or mortality in children who underwent splenectomy. However, they could have more episodes of pain and acute chest syndrome [33].

Total splenectomy prevents the recurrence of splenic sequestration, but there are no clinical trials comparing the efficacy of splenectomy compared to chronic transfusion regimes in patients with SCA.

Total splenectomy in SCA is related to a high risk of fulminant sepsis and increased incidence of other events, which have not been reported in patients with partial splenectomy. Gutiérrez et al. examined 54 patients with SCA, who underwent partial splenectomy and compared the clinical and laboratory results with nonsplenectomized patients. They found that partial splenectomy was a safe procedure in patients with sickle cell disease. There were no differences in the clinical picture in children splenectomized and nonsplenectomized except the greater frequency of hepatic sequestration crisis in the first group [37].

Some authors recommend chronic red cell transfusion to prevent recurrent crises, but this can lead to risks such as hepatitis, HIV, parvovirus, and allosensitization. In addition, many patients developed ASSC when red cell transfusion was stopped [38].

SCA conditions that may require splenectomy are as follows:

a. Recurrent splenic sequestration crisis

b. Discomfort and deterioration in quality of life secondary to hypersplenism and splenomegaly

c. Splenic abscess

d. Massive splenic infarction

e. Splenomegaly with nonfunctioning spleen

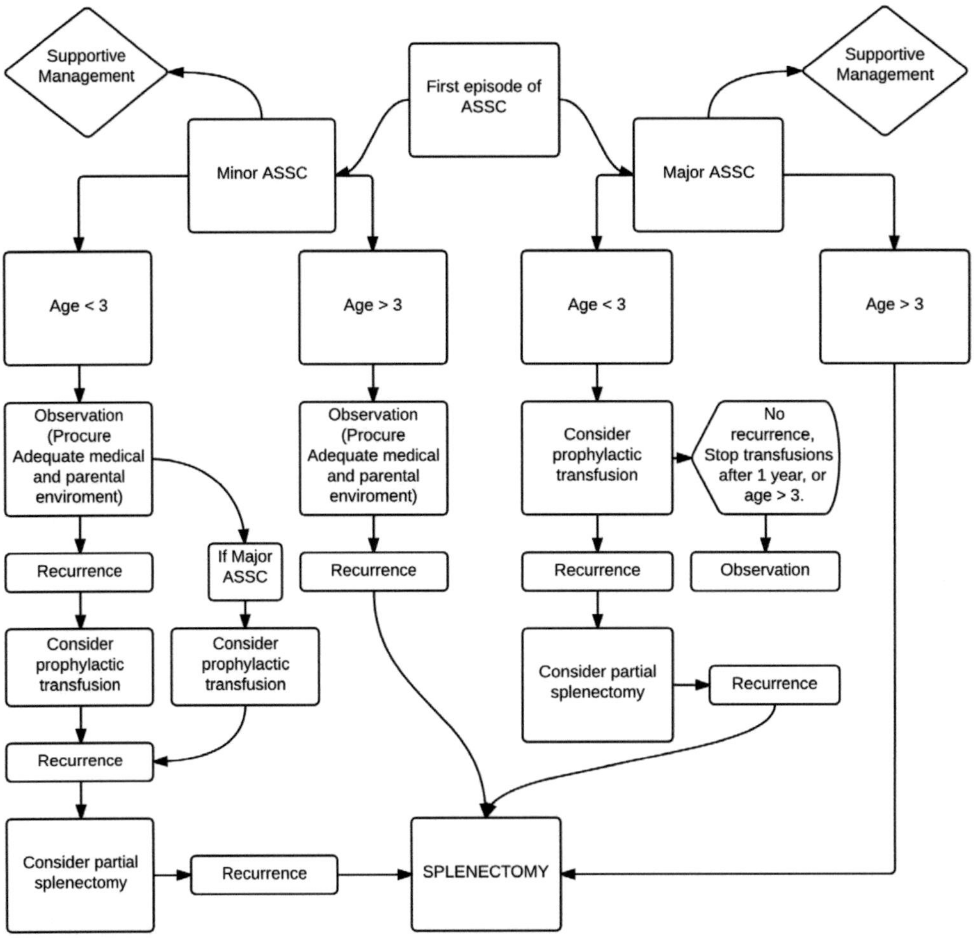

Algorithm 1. Peña and Londoño. Proposed management of ASSC.

5. Follow-up

Patients must be followed periodically, clinically, and with laboratory tests. It is also important to teach the family to palpate the spleen from the diagnosis, warning the need to go quickly to a hospital in case of decay, fever, pallor, and splenomegaly.

Therefore, patients who experience their first ASSC in their first year should be monitored carefully.

Acknowledgements

To our patients who give us lessons of life from day to day.

To Lina Marcela Cadavid Alvarez, MD, Radiologist from Hospital Pablo Tobon Uribe, Medellín, who provided radiological Images.

Author details

Jorge Peña Siado[1*] and Julian Londono Hernández[2]

*Address all correspondence to: penasiado@une.net.co

1 Pediatric Hematologist at Hospital Pablo Tobon Uribe, Medellín, Colombia

2 General Physician at Haematology Service, Fundación Colombiana de Cancerología, Clínica Vida, Medellín, Colombia

References

[1] Herrick J. Peculiar elongated and sickle-shaped red blood corpuscles in a case of severe anemia . Archives of Internal Medicine. 1910;6:517-21.

[2] Ingram VM. A specific chemical difference between the globins of normal human and sickle-cell anaemiahaemoglobin. Nature. 1956;178(4537):792–4.

[3] Lees C, Davies SC, Dezateux C. Neonatal screening for sickle cell disease. Cochrane Database of Systematic Reviews. 2000;(Issue 1):CD001913. DOI: 10.1002/14651858.CD001913.

[4] Brousse V, Buffet P, Rees D. The spleen and sickle cell disease: the sick(led) spleen. British Journal of Haematology. 2014;Jul;166(2):165–76. DOI: 10.1111/bjh.12950

[5] Topley JM, Rogers DW, Stevens MC, Serjeant GR. Acute splenic sequestration and hypersplenism in the first five years in homozygous sickle cell disease. Archives of Disease in Childhood. 1981 Oct;56(10):765–9.

[6] Al-Salem AH. Massive splenic infarction in children with sickle cell anemia and the role of splenectomy. Pediatric Surgery International. 2013 Mar;29(3):281–5. DOI: 10.1007/s00383-012-3223-2.

[7] Al-Salem AH. Indications and complications of splenectomy for children with sickle cell disease. Journal of Pediatric Surgery. 2006 Nov;41(11):1909–15.

[8] Juwah AI, Nlemadim EU, Kaine W. Types of anaemic crises in paediatric patients with sickle cell anaemia seen in Enugu, Nigeria. Archives of Disease in Childhood. 2004 Jun;89(6):572–6.

[9] Poulin EC, Mamazza J, Schlachta CM. Splenic artery embolization before laparoscopic splenectomy. An update. Surgical Endoscopy. Jun 1998;12(6):870–5.

[10] Jeker R. Hypersplenism. TherapeutischeUmschau. 2013 Mar;70(3):152–6. DOI: 10.1024/0040-5930/a000383.

[11] Al-Salem AH. Indications and complications of splenectomy for children with sickle cell disease. Journal of Pediatric Surgery. 2006 Nov;41(11):1909–15.

[12] Kirkineska L, Perifanis V, Vasiliadis T. Functional hyposplenism. Hippokratia. 2014 Jan;18(1):7–11

[13] Di Sabatino A, Carsetti R, Corazza GR. Post-splenectomy and hyposplenic states. Lancet. 2011 Jul 2;378(9785):86–97. DOI: 10.1016/S0140-6736(10)61493-6

[14] Bokman CL, Sfeir M, Chahwala V, Ginzburg E. Spontaneous massive splenic infarction in the setting of renal transplant and septic shock: a case report and review of the literature. Case Reports in Medicine. 2014;2014:510259. DOI: 10.1155/2014/510259.

[15] Airede AI. Acute splenic sequestration in a five-week-old infant with sickle cell disease. Journal of Pediatrics. 1992 Jan;120(1):160.

[16] Emond AM, Collis R, Darvill D, Higgs DR, Maude GH, Serjeant GR. Acute splenic sequestration in homozygous sickle cell disease: natural history and management. Journal of Pediatrics, 1985; 107, 201–6.

[17] Powell RW, Levine GL, Yang YM, Mankad VN. Acute splenic sequestration crisis in sickle cell disease: early detection and treatment. Journal of Pediatric Surgery, 1992; 27, 215–8.

[18] Brousse V, Elie C, Benkerrou M, Odièvre MH, Lesprit E, Bernaudin F, Grimaud M, Guitton C, Quinet B, Dangiolo S, de Montalembert M. Acute splenic sequestration crisis in sickle cell disease: cohort study of 190 paediatric patients. British Journal of Haematology. 2012 Mar;156(5):643–8. DOI: 10.1111/j.1365-2141.2011.08999.x.

[19] William BM, Corazza GR. Hyposplenism: a comprehensive review. Part I: basic concepts and causes. Hematology. 2007;12, 1–13.

[20] Buffet PA, Milon G, Brousse V, Correas JM, Dousset B, Couvelard A, Kianmanesh R, Farges O, Sauvanet A, Paye F, Ungeheuer MN, Ottone C, Khun H, Fiette L, Guigon G, Huerre M, Mercereau-Puijalon O, David PH. Ex vivo perfusion of human spleens maintains clearing and processing functions. Blood. 2006; 107, 3745–52.

[21] Safeukui I, Correas JM, Brousse V, Hirt D, Deplaine G, Mule S, Lesurtel M, Goasguen N, Sauvanet A, Couvelard A, Kerneis S, Khun H, Vigan-Womas I, Ottone C, Molina TJ, Treluyer JM, Mercereau-Puijalon O, Milon G, David PH, Buffet PA. Retention of Plasmodium falciparum ring-infected erythrocytes in the slow, open microcirculation of the human spleen. Blood. 2008; 112, 2520–8.

[22] Donald DE, Aarhus LL. Active and passive release of blood from canine spleen and small intestine. American Journal of Physiology. 1974; 227, 1166–72.

[23] denHaan JM, Kraal G. Innate immune functions of macrophage subpopulations in the spleen. Journal of Innate Immunity. 2012; 4, 437–45.

[24] Bookchin RM, Lew VL. Pathophysiology of sickle cell anemia. Hematology/Oncology Clinics of North America. 1996; 10:1241–53.

[25] Rodgers GP. Overview of pathophysiology and rationale for treatment of sickle cell anemia. Seminars in Hematology. 1997; 34:2–7.

[26] Lonergan GJ, Cline DB, Abbondanz SL. Sickle cell anemia. RadioGraphics. 2001 Jul; 21:971–94,

[27] Mallouh AA, Qudah A. Acute splenic sequestration together with aplastic crisis caused by human parvovirus B19 in patients with sickle cell disease. Journal of Pediatrics. 1993; 122, no. 4, 593–5.

[28] Krishnan S, Setty Y, Betal SG, Vijender V, Rao K, Dampier C, Stuart M. Increased levels of the inflammatory biomarker C-reactive protein at baseline are associated with childhood sickle cell vasocclusive crises. British Journal of Haematology, 2010; 148, 797–804.

[29] Pena S, Velez MC, Sanchez DP, Donado JH. Beneficios de la terapia con hidroxiúrea en niños con anemia de célulasfalciformes. Iatreia [online]. 2012; 25, no. 2, 105–110. ISSN 0121-0793.

[30] Yates AM, Hankins JS, Mortier NA, Aygun B, Ware RE. Simultaneous acute splenic sequestration and transient aplastic crisis in children with sickle cell disease. Pediatric Blood and Cancer. 2009 Sep;53(3):479–81. DOI: 10.1002/pbc.22035

[31] Aneni EC, Hamer DH, Gill CJ. Systematic review of current and emerging strategies for reducing morbidity from malaria in sickle cell disease. Tropical Medicine and International Health. 2013 Mar;18(3):313–27. DOI: 10.1111/tmi.12056.

[32] Harrod VL, Howard TA, Zimmerman SA, Dertinger SD, Ware RE. Quantitative analysis of Howell–Jolly bodies in children with sickle cell disease. Experimental Hematology, 2007; 35, 179–183.

[33] Levin TL, Berdon WE, Haller JO, Ruzal-Shapiro C, Hurlet-Jenson A. Intrasplenic masses of "preserved" functioning splenic tissue in sickle cell disease: correlation of imaging findings (CT, ultrasound, MRI, and nuclear scintigraphy). Pediatric Radiology 1996; 26:646–9.

[34] Josephson CD, Su LL, Hillyer KL, et al. Transfusion in the patient with sickle cell disease: a critical review of the literature and transfusion guidelines. Transfusion Medicine Reviews 2007;21:118–33.

[35] Wright Jg, Hambleton IR, Thomas PW, et al. Postesplenectomy course in homozygous sickle cell disease. Journal of Pediatrics. 1999;134:304–9.

[36] Koduri PR, Nathan S. Acute splenic sequestration crisis in adults with hemoglobin S-C disease: a report of nine cases. Annals of Hematology. 2006;85:239–43.

[37] Gutiérrez Díaz AI, Svarch E, ArencibiaNúñez A, Sabournin Ferrier V, MachínGarcía S, Menendez Veitía A, Ramón Rodriguez L, Serrano Mirabal J, García Peralta T, López Martin LG. Partial splenectomy in sickle cell disease. Anales de Pediatria (Barcelona). 2014 Feb 27. pii: S1695-4033(13)00469-4. DOI: 10.1016/j.anpedi.2013.11.002.

[38] Kinney TR, Ware RE, Schultz WH, et al. Long-term management of splenic sequestration in children with sickle cell disease. Journal of Pediatrics. 1990;117:194–9.

Chapter 6

Comparative Study of the Amount of Re-released Hemoglobin from α-Thalassemia and Hereditary Spherocytosis Erythrocytes

Yan Su, Hongjie Ma, Hongwang Zhang, Lijun Gao,
Guorong Jia, Wenbin Qin and Qitu He

Additional information is available at the end of the chapter

http://dx.doi.org/10.5772/60947

Abstract

Hemoglobin release test (HRT), which is established by our lab, is a new experiment to observe the re-released hemoglobin (Hb) from erythrocytes. In this study, one-dimension HRT, double dimension HRT, and isotonic and hypotonic HRT were performed to observe the re-released Hb from the blood samples of normal adult, hereditary spherocytosis (HS), and α-thalassemia. The results showed that compared with normal adult, the re-released Hb from HS blood sample was decreased significantly; however, the re-released Hb from α-thalassemia blood sample was increased significantly. The mechanism of this phenomenon was speculated to have relation with the abnormal amount of membrane-binding Hb.

Keywords: hereditary spherocytosis, α-thalassemia, hemoglobin release test, erythrocyte, hemoglobin

1. Introduction

Erythrocytes, also called red blood cells (RBCs), are the most common type of blood cell. In humans, mature erythrocytes are flexible and oval biconcave disks. They lack cell nucleus and most organelles, in order to accommodate maximum space for hemoglobin (Hb), which has the important oxygen-transporting function. This protein makes up about 96% of the erythrocytes' dry content (by weight), and around 35% of the total content (including water) [1]. Hb is an assembly of two α-globin family chains (including α and ξ chains) and two β-globin family chains (including β, γ, δ, and ε chains). Each globin subunit has an embedded heme group and each heme group contains an iron atom that can bind one oxygen molecule through iron-induced dipole forces. These subunits are bound to each other by salt bridges, hydrogen bonds, and hydrophobic interactions. Three Hb variants exist in normal adult erythrocytes, that is HbA ($\alpha_2\beta_2$, over 95%), HbF ($\alpha_2\gamma_2$, <1%), and HbA_2 ($\alpha_2\delta_2$, 1.5–3.5%) [2-3].

The erythrocyte membrane plays many roles that aid in regulating erythrocytes' surface deformability, flexibility, adhesion to other cells, and immune recognition. These functions are highly dependent on the composition of the membrane, which includes 3 layers: the glycocalyx on the exterior, which is rich in carbohydrates; the lipid bilayer, which contains many transmembrane proteins, besides its lipidic main constituents; and the membrane skeleton, a structural network of proteins located on the inner surface of the lipid bilayer. The determinant of normal membrane cohesion is the system of "vertical" linkages between the phospholipid bilayer and membrane skeleton, formed by the interactions of the cytoplasmic domains of various membrane proteins with the spectrin-based skeletal network. Band 3 and Rh-associated glycoprotein (RhAG) provide such links by interacting with ankyrin, which in turn binds to β-spectrin. Protein 4.2 binds to both band 3 and ankyrin and can regulate the avidity of the interaction between band 3 and ankyrin. Glycophorin C, band 3, XK, Rh, and Duffy all bind to protein 4.1R, the third member of the ternary junctional complex with β-spectrin and actin [4].

Thalassemia is an inherited autosomal recessive blood disorder characterized by abnormal formation of Hb, which results in improper oxygen transport and destruction of erythrocytes. Normally, the majority of adult Hb (HbA), is composed of two α- and two β-globin chains, which are arranged into a heterotetramer. The β-globin chain is encoded by a single gene on chromosome 11 [5], and α-globin chain is encoded by two closely linked genes on chromosome 16 [6]. A normal person has two loci encoding the β-chain, and four loci encoding the α-chain. Thalassemia patients have defects in either the α- or β-globin chain. According to which chain is affected, thalassemias are classified into α-thalassemias and β-thalassemia. α-thalassemias result in decreased α-globin production, which result in an excess of β-chains in adults and excess γ-chains in newborns. The excess β-globin chains form unstable tetramers (HbH, β_4), which have abnormal oxygen dissociation curves. β-thalassemias are characterized as either β^o or β-thalassemia major if formation of any β chains is prevented, the most severe form of β-thalassemia; as either β^+ or β thalassemia intermedia if some β-globin chain formation are allowed; or as β-thalassemia minor if β-globin chain production is not terribly compromised [7-8]. In contrast to the β-thalassemias, which are usually caused by point mutations of the β-globin gene, the α-thalassemia syndromes are usually caused by the deletion of one or more α-globin genes and are subclassified according to the number of α-globin genes that are deleted (or mutated): one gene deleted (α^+-thalassemia); two genes deleted on the same chromosome or in cis (α^0-thalassemia); three genes deleted (HbH disease); or four genes deleted (hydrops fetalis with Hb Bart's) [8].

Hereditary spherocytosis (HS) is an autosomal dominant erythrocyte membranopathy [9], but does not belong to hereditary hemoglobinopathies. This disorder is caused by mutations in genes relating to membrane proteins. These proteins include spectrin (α and β), ankyrin [10], band 3, protein 4.2 [11], and other erythrocyte membrane proteins that allow for the erythrocytes to change their shapes. The abnormal erythrocytes are sphere-shaped (spherocytosis) rather than being the normal biconcave disk shaped. This difference in shape not only interferes with the ability to be flexible to travel from the arteries to the smaller capillaries, but also makes the erythrocytes more prone to rupture.

Hemoglobin release test (HRT), also called electrophoresis release test (ERT), which is performed by electrophoresing live erythrocytes directly on a starch–agarose mixed gel with intermittent electric current, was established by our lab in 2007 [3,12]. Starch–agarose mixed gel electrophoresis is a routine method used to separate and analyze Hb in our lab since 1980. Hb within the erythrocytes can only be released once during routine starch–agarose mixed gel electrophoresis, which is performed with continuous power supply, and this phenomenon is named as "initial release" now. The difference in mobility of HbA_2 between erythrocyte and hemolysate sample (also called HbA_2 phenomenon) was found during an "initial release" experiment in 1981 [12]. In 2007, a sudden power outage was encountered during the electrophoresis of erythrocytes, however, the experiment was not abandoned and electrophoresis was continued after the power was restored. To our surprise, another new Hb band was found to be released from the origin, which was named "single-band re-release" as opposed to the "initial release". When the power outages were simulated more than once, multiple Hb bands would appear between HbA and origin, and this phenomenon was named as multiple-band re-release or ladder-band re-release [13]. Based on these experiments, isotonic and hypotonic HRT and double-dimensional HRT were developed subsequently. Then the re-released Hb was observed in many patients' erythrocytes, and its amount varied in different patients [14-15]. Some of the patients had increased Hb re-release, such as β-thalassemia, some general surgery patients, cirrhosis, and some gastro enteric tumor patients, but the specific screening experiment had not been done and the exact mechanism of this phenomenon had not been clear. The erythrocyte membrane or cytoskeleton binding Hb was speculated to have relationship with this phenomenon. To further study the mechanism of Hb re-release, the effects of blood type, blood viscosity, different membrane-destroying methods, exogenous hydrogen peroxide, and glutaraldehyde treatments on the amount of re-released Hb were observed subsequently, and the re-released Hb was speculated to have relationship with the abnormality of erythrocyte membrane and Hb. In this study, re-released Hb from two hereditary hemolytic diseases, HS (erythrocyte membrane disorder) and α-thalassemia (Hb disorder), was observed with a variety of HRT experiments.

2. The comparative study of the re-released hemoglobin from α-thalassemia and hereditary spherocytosis erythrocytes

This study had been approved by the local ethics committee, and one HS patient (coming from the first hospital of Baotou Medical College) and one α- thalassemia patient (coming from the third Worker's Hospital of Baogang Group) were included. The HS patient, diagnosed as spectrin defect, is a 45-year-old female with hemolytic anemia, jaundice, and splenomegaly. The α- thalassemia patient, diagnosed as Southeast Asian deletion (SEA) by PCR, is a 35-year-old female with hemolytic anemia and splenomegaly. Before collecting their blood, patients were asked to sign the consent information. Venous blood samples were anticoagulated with EDTA, and then routine blood examination, osmotic fragility test and HRT were performed respectively within 24 h. The spherical erythrocytes of HS patient are more than 20% in peripheral blood smear, and the osmotic fragility is increased (max: 0.39% vs 0.40%-0.45%, min: 0.75% vs 0.55%-0.6%). As to the α-thalassemia patient, a large number of target erythrocytes exist in peripheral blood smear and the osmotic fragility is decreased.

Whole blood was divided into two parts, one part was used to prepare blood samples, and the other part was used to prepare RBC samples. Blood samples were prepared by adding the same volume of CCl_4 into the anticoagulated blood. After turbulent mixing and centrifuging (12000 rpm for 10 minutes), the upper layer was whole blood hemolysate, the middle layer between hemolysate and CCl_4 was whole blood stroma. The other part of whole blood was firstly made into packed RBCs by washing the RBCs with saline for 4-5 times until the supernatant was colorless [3,12,13]. Then the same volume of CCl_4 was added into the packed RBCs, and after mixing and centrifuging (3000 rpm for 10 minutes), the upper red solution was RBC hemolysate, and the middle layer between hemolysate and CCl_4 was RBC stroma.

The starch–agarose mixed gel was prepared by dissolving 0.24 g of agarose and 1.72 g of starch in 90 mL of TEB buffer (42.1 mmol/L Tris, 1.71 mmol/L EDTA, 6.47 mmol/L boric acid, pH 8.6) [3,12,13]. The solution was heated until the agarose melts, and then the gel was laid on a 17×17 cm glass while hot. After solidification, about 8 μL of samples were applied on the cathodic side of the gel by using 3 MM filter paper. After adding blood samples on the starch–agarose mixed gel, electrophoresis was carried out in borate buffer (0.3 mol/L boracic acid, 0.06 mol/L NaOH, pH9.0) at 5 V/cm for 2 hours, then paused for 15 minutes and ran for 15 minutes by turns. It took about 6 hours for the entire electrophoresis. After electrophoresis, the red bands on the gel were firstly observed directly with eyes, and then the gel was sequentially stained with Ponceau Red (0.1% Ponceau S, 5% glacial acetic acid and 2% glycerol) and Benzidine (0.6 g of benzidine, 25 mL of glacial acetic acid, 10 mL of glycerol, add deionized water to 500 mL, then keep the solution in 75℃ water bath for 1 hour until the benzidine is dissolved completely. Sodium nitroprusside and 30% H_2O_2 should be added to this solution before use) for 4 hours, respectively. Finally, the gel was rinsed with rinsing solution (5% glacial acetic acid, 2% glycerin) until the background was clear.

Routine one-directional HRT was performed to compare the re-released Hb from normal, α-thalassemia, and HS patients' blood samples, which were prepared from whole blood, whole blood hemolysate, whole blood stroma, RBCs, RBCs hemolysate, RBCs stroma and plasma respectively. Comparing with the normal control, the re-released Hb from HS and α-thalassemia erythrocytes had opposite changes (Figure 1). In normal control, there was nearly no HbA in the sample of whole blood stroma, but a small amount of HbA in the RBCs stroma; both whole blood and RBCs sample of normal control had re-released Hb; however re-released Hb did not appear in whole blood and RBCs hemolysate samples. As to HS, there was more

HbA appearing in RBCs stroma sample, and no re-released Hb appeared in any of the blood samples. On the contrary, the HbA of α-thalassemia whole blood stroma increased significantly, but that of α-thalassemia RBCs stroma was hard to see; in addition, the re-released Hb from whole blood and RBCs sample of α-thalassemia were increased significantly and Hb ladder was formed obviously.

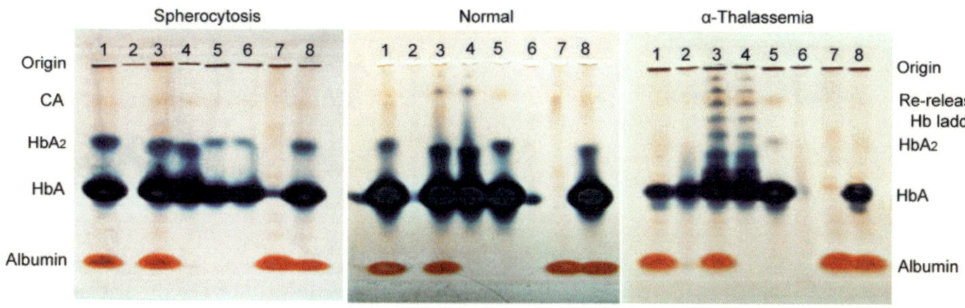

Figure 1. One dimension HRT of spherocytosis and α-thalassemia blood samples. Samples 1–8 were whole blood hemolysate, whole blood stroma, whole blood, RBCs, RBCs hemolysate, RBCs stroma, plasma, whole blood hemolysate.

To observe the effect of hypotonic treatment on the re-released Hb, isotonic and hypotonic HRT was performed with normal adult, HS patient, and α-thalassemia patient at room temperature or 37℃ for 1 hour. During the experiment, the whole blood or packed RBCs were firstly diluted with H_2O in the proportion from 10: 0 to 1: 9 (named as tube 1 to 10, respectively), and then kept at room temperature or 37℃ for 1 hour. Then one-direction HRT was performed as described above. The result of room temperature isotonic and hypotonic HRT showed that the whole blood sample (tube 1) of normal control had slight ladder of re-released Hb, when diluted with H_2O (tube 2 to tube 5), the re-released Hb was decreased, but increased from tube 6 to tube 8, and then decreased again from tube 9 (Figure 2). Compared with the normal control, the re-released Hb ladder decreased obviously in the HS patient, but increased significantly in the α-thalassemia patient. (Figure 2).

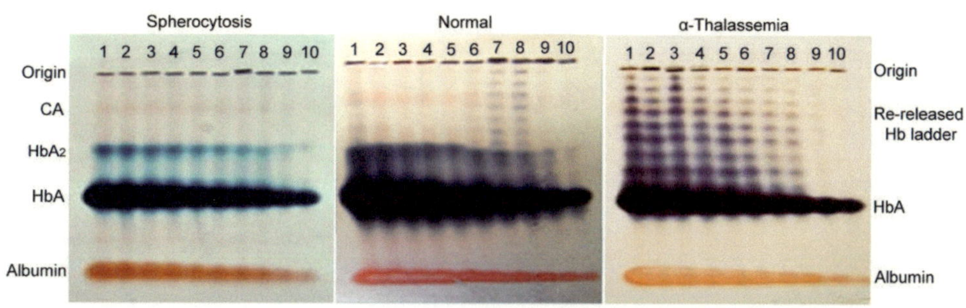

Figure 2. Whole blood isotonic and hypotonic HRT results of normal adult, spherocytosis, and α-thalassemia at room temperature. Whole blood was diluted with H_2O in the proportion from 10: 0 to 1: 9, respectively (tube 1 to 10), and kept at room temperature for 1 hour.

The result (Figure 3) of 37℃ isotonic and hypotonic HRT was similar with that at room temperature except for the disappearance of re-released Hb ladder from tube 1 of the normal control.

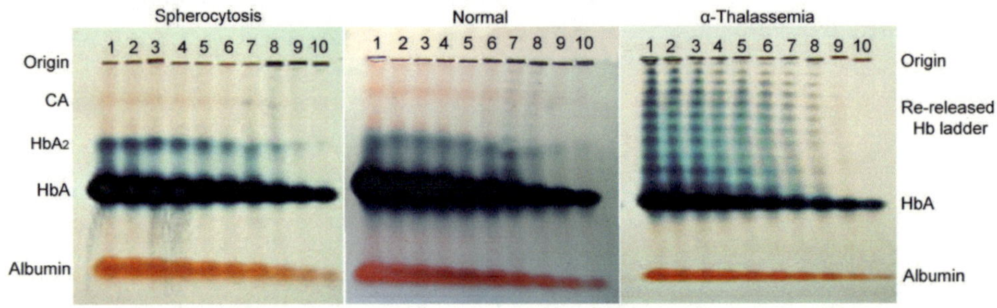

Figure 3. Whole blood isotonic and hypotonic HRT results of normal adult, spherocytosis, and α-thalassemias at 37℃. Whole blood was diluted with H2O in the proportion from 10: 0 to 1: 9, respectively (tube 1 to 10), and kept at 37℃ for 1 hour.

Double-direction HRT (or diagonal HRT) was performed to observe not only the re-released HbA but also the re-released HbA_2. Firstly, one-direction HRT was performed as described above, then the direction of electric field was changed vertical to the original one, and another cycle of HRT was performed. The result showed that there was few re-released HbA in normal whole blood, but the re-released HbA_2 was difficult to observe (Figure 4A). Compared with normal, the re-released HbA from HS whole blood was decreased, but that from α-thalassemia whole blood was increased significantly. The amount of HbA_2 in α-thalassemia whole blood was less than the normal control obviously, and the re-released HbA_2 could not be detected in our experiment (Figure 4B).

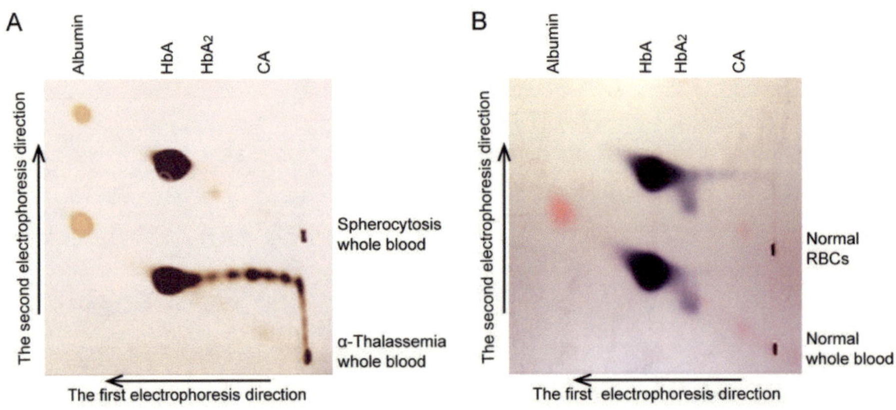

Figure 4. Double-direction HRT of normal adult, spherocytosis, and α-thalassemias blood sample. A was the double-direction HRT of spherocytosis and α-thalassemia whole blood sample; B was the double-direction HRT of the normal whole blood and RBCs sample.

http://dx.doi.org/10.5772/60947

3. Discussion

Both HS and thalassemia belong to hereditary hemolytic disorders, which include hemoglobinopathies, erythrocyte membranopathy, and erythrocyte enzymopathy [16]. HS is the representative erythrocyte membranopathy [17], and thalassemia is the classic hemoglobinopathy [18-20]. In this study, Clinical tests showed that anemia, splenomegaly, and jaundice were the common clinical signs and symptoms of these two patients [16]. Some of the erythrocytes of the HS patient were spherical, but that of α-thalassemia were target-shaped. The osmotic fragility of erythrocytes increased in HS, but decreased in α-thalassemia. The morphology and osmotic fragility changes were caused by the defects of these two disorders. The abnormalities in HS erythrocyte membrane proteins, particularly ankyrin, α- and β-spectrin, band 3 and protein 4.2, result in the loss of membrane surface area relative to intracellular volume, which leads to spherically shaped erythrocytes with decreased deformability and increased fragility. Increased erythrocyte fragility leads to vesiculation and further membrane loss [21], so HS erythrocytes are unable to withstand the introduction of small amounts of free water that occurs when they are placed in increasingly hypotonic saline solutions. As a consequence, HS erythrocytes hemolyze more readily than normal erythrocytes at any saline concentration [17].

The thalassemic erythrocyte membranes exhibit morphological, biochemical, and mechanical abnormalities due to oxidative damage induced by binding of unmatched globin chains to the cytoplasmic surface of the membrane. So both α- and β- thalassemic erythrocytes become renitent and are less deformable than normal erythrocytes. The morphology and mechanical properties of the erythrocytes membrane are controlled by the cytoskeletal network underlying the lipid bilayer. Spectrin is the principal structural element of the erythrocyte cytoskeleton, regulating membrane cytoskeletal functions [22].

The re-released Hb was compared between these two kinds of hereditary hemolytic disorders by HRT. The results showed that comparing with the normal control, the re-released Hb from HS whole blood or erythrocytes was decreased, but increased distinctively from that of α-thalassemic erythrocytes during routine, two-directional, and isotonic and hypotonic HRT. The re-released Hb is speculated to have relationship with membrane-binding Hb, and the abnormal membrane-binding Hb will lead to abnormal Hb re-release. As known, most of the Hb exists in cytoplasm; only small amount of Hb binds with the membrane through interaction with the cytoskeletal proteins or membrane lipids. The abnormality of both membrane and Hb will change the amount of membrane-binding Hb, and will further lead to the variation of re-released Hb during HRT. HRT was established by our lab in 2007, and in the previous studies, the re-released Hb usually increased from some patients' erythrocytes during HRT, such as β-thalassemia patients, some general surgery patients, cirrhosis, and some gastroenteric tumor patients. In our study, the re-released Hb from α-thalassemic erythrocytes was increased significantly like before [12], but the re-released Hb from HS erythrocytes was decreased a lot. The abnormal membrane-binding Hb was speculated to be the reason.

It is well known that in vivo and under normal physiological conditions, intraerythrocytic hemoglobin may exist in three different forms represented by oxygenated, deoxygenated and partially oxidized Hb. Apart from the first two derivatives whose relative proportions are continuously changing during the oxygenation deoxygenation cycle, met-hemoglobin (MetHb) is normally present at a steady-state level of about 1% [23]. MetHb usually binds with membrane, and the re-released Hb from normal erythrocytes is speculated to be the membrane-binding MetHb. Oxidative damage can lead to the oxidative membrane damage and increased proportion of MetHb. The oxidization of band 3 leads to dissociation of ankyrin from band 3, and then tetrameric MetHb cross-link with the cytoplasmic domain of oxidized band 3 dimer [24]. In addition to MetHb, the abnormal Hb in all kinds of hemoglobinopathies is speculated to be the other main source of re-released Hb. α-thalassemia has the defect in α-globin syntheses, the relative excess of β-globin increases and the abnormal HbH (β_4) forms, which can bind with the membrane and lead to the increased Hb re-release.

Hb usually has interaction with spectrin, and the spectrin defect in HS patient interfere the binding of Hb with membrane, so the membrane-binding Hb and re-released Hb decreased obviously. There are five main kinds of erythrocyte skeleton proteins; defect of different cytoskeletal protein might leads to different results.

In conclusion, the change of re-released Hb is only an experimental phenomenon of HRT, and the mechanism of HRT has not been clear very much. In the future, more and more studies are needed to clarify these.

Acknowledgements

This work was supported by grants from Natural Science Foundation of China (81160214), Major Projects of Higher Education Scientific Research in the Inner Mongolia Autonomous Region (NJ09157), Key Science and Technology Research Project of the Ministry of Education, Natural Science Foundation of Inner Mongolia (2010BS1101). We also especially acknowledge all of the people who donated their blood samples for our research.

Author details

Yan Su[1], Hongjie Ma[2], Hongwang Zhang[3], Lijun Gao[1], Guorong Jia[2], Wenbin Qin[1*] and Qitu He[2*]

*Address all correspondence to: qinwenbinbt@sohu.com; Heqitu@163.com

1 Laboratory of Hemoglobin, Baotou Medical College, Baotou, China

2 Department of Hematology, the First Affiliated Hospital of Baotou Medical College, Baotou, China

3 Clinical Laboratory, the third Worker's Hospital of Baogang Group, Baotou, China

Yan Su and Hongjie Ma contribute equally to this work.

References

[1] Weed RI, Reed CF, Berg G. Is hemoglobin an essential structural component of human erythrocyte membranes? The Journal of Clinical Investigation. 1963;42:581-588.

[2] Ribeil JA, Arlet JB, Dussiot M, Moura IC, Courtois G, Hermine O. Ineffective erythropoiesis in β -thalassemia. Scientific World Journal. 2013;2013:394295. DOI: 10.1155/2013/394295.

[3] Su Y, Gao L, Ma Q, Zhou L, Qin L, Han L, Qin W. Interactions of hemoglobin in live red blood cells measured by the electrophoresis release test. Electrophoresis. 2010;31(17):2913-2920. DOI : 10.1002/elps.201000034.

[4] Barcellini W, Bianchi P, Fermo E, Imperiali FG, Marcello AP, Vercellati C, Zaninoni A, Zanella A. Hereditary red cell membrane defects: diagnostic and clinical aspects. Blood Transfusion. 2011;9(3):274-277.

[5] Schwartz E, Cohen A, Surrey S. Overview of the beta thalassemias: genetic and clinical aspects. Hemoglobin. 1988;12(5-6):551-564.

[6] Bernini LF, Harteveld CL. Alpha-thalassaemia. Bailliere's Clinical Haematology. 1998;11(1):53-90.

[7] Clarke GM, Higgins TN. Laboratory investigation of hemoglobinopathies and thalassemias: review and update. Clinical Chemistry. 2000;46(8 Pt 2):1284-1290.

[8] Forget BG, Bunn HF. Classification of the Disorders of Hemoglobin. Cold Spring Harb Perspect Med. 2013;3:a011684. DOI: 10.1101/cshperspect.a011684.

[9] Guitton C, Garçon L, Cynober T, Gauthier F, Tchernia G, Delaunay J, Leblanc T, Thuret I, Bader-Meunier B. Hereditary spherocytosis: guidelines for the diagnosis and management in children. Archives de Pediatrie. 2008;15(9):1464-1473. DOI: 10.1016/j.

[10] Gallagher PG, Forget BG. Hematologically important mutations: spectrin and ankyrin variants in hereditary spherocytosis. Blood Cells, Molecules and Diseases. 1998;24(4):539-543.

[11] Perrotta S, Gallagher PG, Mohandas N. Hereditary spherocytosis. Lancet. 2008;372(9647):1411-1426. DOI:10.1016/S0140-6736(08)61588-3.

[12] Su Y, Shao G, Gao L, Zhou L, Qin L, Qin W. RBC electrophoresis with discontinuous power supply - a newly established hemoglobin release test. Electrophoresis. 2009;30(17):3041-3043. DOI: 10.1002/elps.200900176.

[13] Su Y, Shen J, Gao L, Tian Z, Tian H, Qin L, Qin W. Molecular Interactions of Re-released proteins in Electrophoresis of Human Erythrocytes. Electrophoresis. 2012;33 (9-10): 1402-1405. DOI: 10.1002/elps.201100644.

[14] Qin W. Electrophoresis release of hemoglobin from living red blood cells. Scientia Sinica(Vitae). 2014;41(8):597-607.

[15] Li JX, Su Y. Clinical research progress of red cell hemoglobin release test. Progress in Veterinary Medicine. 2014;35(10):104-107.

[16] Dhaliwal G, Cornett PA, Tierney LM Jr. Hemolytic anemia. American Academy of Family Physicians. 2004;69(11):2599-2606.

[17] Gallagher PG. Abnormalities of the erythrocyte membrane. Pediatric Clinic of North America. 2013;60(6):1349-1362. DOI: 10.1016/j.pcl.2013.09.001.

[18] De Franceschi L, Bertoldi M, Matte A, Santos Franco S, Pantaleo A, Ferru E, Turrini F. Oxidative stress and β-thalassemic erythroid cells behind the molecular defect. Oxidative Medicine and Cellular Longevity. 2013;2013:985210. DOI: 10.1155/2013/985210.

[19] Modell B, Darlison M. Global epidemiology of haemoglobin disorders and derived service indicators. Bulletin of the World Health Organization. 2008;86(6):480-487.

[20] Weatherall DJ. The global problem of genetic disease. Annals of Human Biology. 2005;32(2):117-122.

[21] Alaarg A, Schiffelers RM, van Solinge WW, van Wijk R. Red blood cell vesiculation in hereditary hemolytic anemia. Frontiers of Physiology. 2013;4(365):1-82. DOI: 10.3389/fphys.

[22] Rutaiwan T, Pornpimol M, Prapon W. Status of red cell membrane protein phosphorylation in thalassemia. ScienceAsia-Journal of the Science Society of Thailand. 2002;28: 313-317.

[23] Giardina B, Scatena R, Clementi ME, Ramacci MT, Maccari F, Cerroni L, Condò SG. Selective binding of met-hemoglobin to erythrocytic membrane: a possible involvement in red blood cell aging. Advances in Experimental Medicine and Biology. 1991;307:75-84.

[24] Arashiki N, Kimata N, Manno S, Mohandas N, Takakuwa Y. Membrane peroxidation and methemoglobin formation are both necessary for band 3 clustering: mechanistic insights into human erythrocyte senescence. Biochemistry. 2013;52(34):5760-5769. DOI: 10.1021/bi400405p.

Section 2

Therapeutic Strategies

Chapter 7

Modifiers of γ-Globin Gene Expression and Treatment of β-Thalassemia

Anjana Munshi, Sneha Dadeech, M. Sai Babu and Preeti Khetarpal

Additional information is available at the end of the chapter

http://dx.doi.org/10.5772/61441

Abstract

Beta thalassemia (β-thalassemia) is an autosomal recessive genetic disease with many genes involved. It is a heterogeneous disorder caused by variations in the inactivation mechanism of the Beta-globin (β-globin) genes. Despite seemingly similar genotypes, the patients with Beta-thalassemia have a remarkable variability in anaemia, growth development, and hepatospleenomegaly and transfusion requirements. The genetic factors may differ in each race or ethnic group for therapy and prevention. Despite remarkable successes in the treatment of Beta-thalassemia in the past decades, it is still the leading cause of death and premature disability in developed and developing countries. Possible factors that influence the severity of anaemia in thalassemia may be inherited or non-inherited. The inherited factors include the type of β-thalassemia, coinheritance of alpha thalassemia (α-thalassemia) and factors that stimulate fetal hemoglobin (HbF) production. In this chapter, respective contributions of known modifiers and also the pharmaceutical agents currently in use and under clinical trials for regulating the globin gene expression will be discussed.

Keywords: Hemoglobinopathies, gamma globin, fetal hemoglobin, modifier genes, drug discovery

1. Introduction

1.1. General introduction

The thalassemias are the commonest monogenic disorders in the world, and globally it is estimated that there are 270 million carriers, of which 80 million are carriers of β-thalassemia. β-thalassemia is widespread in the Mediterranean, Southeast Asian, African, and Middle East populations. The mean prevalence of this disease in India is 3.3%. It has become much more common recently in northern and central Europe, including Germany, due to immigration [1–

3]. The thalassemias refer to a diverse group of hemoglobin disorders characterized by a reduced synthesis of one or more of the globin chains (α, β, γ, δβ, γδβ, δ, and εγδβ). β-thalassemia occurs when there is a deficiency of β-globin, which is typically caused by a direct down-regulation in the synthesis of structurally normal b chains. However, a thalassemia phenotype can also arise from structural b chain variants if they are synthesized at a reduced rate. The most severe form of thalassemias is characterized by the complete absence of HbA ($\alpha_2\beta_2$) which results from the inheritance of two homozygous β-thalassemia alleles. This normally presents as a life-threatening anemia requiring blood transfusions from infancy. Inheritance of single β-thalassemia alleles is presented by a clinically asymptomatic condition, but may show a mild anemia [4].

More than 200 mutations of the β-globin gene which can lead to β-thalassemia major have been characterized worldwide [5–8]. Deletion mutations are rare; the majority of mutations are point mutations in important functional regions of the β-globin gene [9]. Splice mutations and those that occur in the promoter region tend to cause a reduction, rather than a complete absence of β-globin chains, and thus result in milder disease. Nonsense mutations and frameshift mutations tend not to produce any β-globin chains leading to severe disease (loss of function). The severity of anemia caused by β-thalassemia depends on which mutations are present and on whether they decrease beta-globin production (called $beta^+$ thalassemia) or there is complete elimination (called $beta^0$ thalassemia). A subset of common mutations is present in each ethnic group in which the disease is prevalent.

2. Clinical heterogenity in β-thalassemia

Clinical manifestations of β-thalassemia are extremely variable, ranging from nearly asymptomatic to severe and transfusion-dependant [10]. However, the marked variability of the clinical manifestations is not well-understood till date. The clinical picture in some patients may be a devastating course of acute and chronic events, resulting in severe organ damage. In other patients, the disease may be present with relatively mild clinical phenotype and minimal morbidity [11].

3. Factors influencing clinical severity

Various factors have been found to modulate the beta-thalassemia phenotype. These include the presence of alpha-thalassemia, elevated HbF levels, haplotypes that are linked to the beta-globin gene and chromosomal sites different from chromosome 11 [12]. Co-inheritance of a single alpha-globin (α-globin) gene deletion with β-thalassemia may have a milder phenotype, whereas deletion of both α-globin genes is typically associated with thalassemia intermedia [13]. Fetal hemoglobin is one of the most common and major modifiers of the disease severity in individuals with β-thalassemia. Because the severity of homozygous β-thalassemia is directly related to the imbalance between α- and β-globin chains, even the low levels of γ-

http://dx.doi.org/10.5772/61441

globin in F cells reduce the relative excess of α-globin and provide a selective survival of cells making HbF at the time of ineffective erythropoiesis, in the most severe forms of β-thalassemia. Any factor that can reduce the degree of imbalance (by reducing α or increasing β and/or γ globin chains) may ameliorate the clinical phenotype [14]. Therefore, this selective survival might account for elevated levels of HbF in homozygous β-thalassemia. The presence of genetic variants that sustained fetal hemoglobin production have a strong impact on ameliorating the clinical phenotype.

4. Elevated levels of fetal hemoglobin (HbF)

HbF ($\alpha_2\gamma_2$) accounts for up to 90% of the total hemoglobin at birth. Its synthesis starts to decline during the third trimester, and over the first year of life, it is gradually replaced by adult Hb ($\alpha_2\beta_2$). An elevated level of HbF in an adult may result from a genetic disorder of hemoglobin production or from various acquired hematological conditions (such as placental insufficiency) in newborn infants of diabetic mothers, such as severe anemia, bronchopulmonary dysplasia (BPD), and congenital cyanotic heart (CCHD) [15–18]. Erythropoietic stress and hypoxemia has also been shown to increase the production of HbF [19–21]. Additional γ-globin chains bind with the excess of α-chains and decrease the imbalance between α- and β-globin chains caused because of absence of beta-globin chains, decreasing the deleterious effect of intracellular precipitation of unbound β-chains [22–23]. This reduces ineffective erythropoiesis and some functional HbF is produced in the red cell precursors which help red blood cells survive longer duration in the circulation. Induction of fetal haemoglobin expression in erythroid cells is an important therapeutic approach in patients with haemoglobin disease [24-25].

5. Genetic modifiers of γ-globin gene expression

To understand the clinical or molecular relationships, it is important to remember that the main pathophysiological determinant of the severity of beta-thalassemia is more than that of alpha/non-alpha-globin chain imbalance. Therefore, any factor capable of reducing the alpha/non-alpha-globin chain imbalance may have an ameliorating effect on the clinical picture [7]. Certain mutations within the β-globin promoter region are associated with increased γ-chain expression from the same chromosome [7]. These are known as primary modifiers. Recently, genetic variants that modulate HbF levels, but fall outside of the Hb genes (Secondary modifiers) have also been identified [26]. These modifiers, known as secondary modifiers, primarily act directly to alter the known pathophysiology of the disease.

5.1. Primary modifiers

Primary modifiers have been identified as different mutations within the β-globin gene resulting in varying severity. Severity of β-thalassemia ranges from the mutations (β0) causing complete absence of β-globin production to those in which β-globin is produced but to a small extent (β+). Inheritance of two β+ genes such as -28 ATA box (A → G) codon 19 (A → G); -90

C → T, -88 C → A; -88 C → T, -87 C → A; -87 C → G, -87 C → T; -86 C → G, 31 A → G results in a milder disease [27].

Some β-thalassemia mutations are completely silent and have been shown to cause a milder form of the disease. The most common is the -101 (C → T) mutation which interacts with different severe β-thalassemia alleles to produce a mild form of the disease [28]. Co-inheritance of severe β-thalassemia allele (β^0) with hemoglobin E (HbE) allele also results in variability of the phenotype. Alternative to the splicing of HbE globin pre-mRNA, the amount of mRNA spliced may also play a role in the phenotypic variability.

5.2. Secondary modifiers

Secondary genetic modifiers affect the clinical severity of the disease by reducing the globin chain imbalance, therefore resulting in a milder form of the disease phenotype [29]. Genome-wide studies (GWAS) have shown the association of genetic polymorphisms in three major loci Xmn1-HBG2, HBS1L-MYB intergenic region (HMIP) on chromosome 6q23, and BCL11A on chromosome 2p16, accountable for a relatively large proportion of the phenotypic variation in HbF levels. The gene encoding for zinc fingers and homeobox 2 (ZHX2) transcription factor located on 8q24 has emerged as a potential candidate gene for γ-globin regulation.

- Xmn-1 (Xanthomonas maniholis-1) Restriction Site

The presence of one polymorphism Xmn-1 restriction site at -158 position of the Gγ gene has been co-related with the increased production of HbF in adults under haematopoietic stress. A specific (C → T) mutation at the -158 position in the promoter region of the Gγ gene creates a restriction site for the Xmn-1 endonuclease. Higher expression of the fetal hemoglobin (HbF) in adulthood has been indicated to ameliorate the morbidity and mortality in sickle cell disease (SCD). Nemati et al. have studied the frequency of Xmn1 polymorphic sites in β-thalassemia major patients from Western Iran. The study revealed that the presence of this polymorphic site caused a positive influence on HbF production and the G-γ percent, which could improve the clinical symptoms of β-thalassemia patients [30]. In another study carried out by Pandey et al., the phenotypes of Indian sickle cell patients were found to be greatly influenced by Xmn1polymorphism [31].

In a recent study, we have evaluated the association of Xmn1 polymorphism with mild, moderate, and severe groups of β-thalassemia as well as sickle cell anemia (SCA). A significant association of TT genotype and T allele was observed with milder disease phenotype. In addition, we also evaluated the association of Xmn1 polymorphism with HbF levels to estimate whether this variant modifies the phenotype of homozygous β-thalassemia as well as SCA by modulating the HbF levels. A significant difference in the high and low percentage of HbF in CC, CT, and TT bearing individuals ($P<0.01$) were observed. This study confirms that increased γG-globin expression, associated with the Xmn1 polymorphism ameliorates the clinical severity in β-thalassemia as well as SCA in the study population [32].

- Zinc-fingers and homeoboxes 2 (ZHX2) gene

The gene coding for ZHX2 or KIAA0854 in human is located on chromosome 8q24.13 in the position 123863082-124055936. Four exons code for 837 amino acid protein of approximately

http://dx.doi.org/10.5772/61441

92 kDa. The ZHX2 mRNA is expressed among various tissues. ZHX2 is a transcriptional repressor [33] and has been identified as a factor which is involved in postnatal repression of fetal expressing genes [34]. Therefore, ZHX2 is a novel candidate gene for globin regulation in erythroid cells [35]. In 2005, Perencheri et al. indicated that overexpression of a ZHX2 transgene restores H19 repression on a BALB/cj background, confirming that this gene is responsible for hereditary persistence of the α-fetoprotein (Afp) and H19 which are transcribed at high levels in the mammalian fetal liver but are rapidly repressed postnatally [36]. Down-regulation of ZHX2 was recently demonstrated in two HPFH-2 subjects by real-time PCR [35].

ZHX2 gene coincides on the quantitative trait loci (QTL) on chromosome 8q that has been reported to influence the absolute fetalhemoglobin levels [37]. Taken together, ZHX2 is a good candidate gene for regulating γ-globin gene expression. Aussara Panya et al. demonstrated the effect of ZHX2 overexpression and the down-regulation of γ-globin expression in K562 cells [38]. Further, their study supported that ZHX2 is involved in the repression of the γ-globin gene, but also provides evidence that ZHX2 has a direct effect on the γ-globin expression level and might participate in the globin gene regulation [38]. In another study, de Andrade et al. reported the marked down-regulation of ZHX2 in CD34+ cells cultured in a high fetalhemoglobin-enriched condition [39].

- B-cell lymphoma/leukemia 11A (BCL11A) Gene

The BCL11A gene is essential for normal lymphoid development [40] and has been associated with hematologic malignancies [41]. The BCL11A gene was initially identified from aberrant chromosomal translocations involving the immunoglobulin-heavy chain locus detected in B-cell non-Hodgkin lymphomas [42]. It encodes a kruppel-link zinc finger protein containing 3 C_2H_2 zinc finger motifs, a proline-rich region, and an acidic domain. BCL11A gene located on chromosome 2p16.1 is expressed predominantly in the brain, spleen, and testis.

A study has demonstrated that an intronic SNP in BCL11A, rs11886868 strongly co-relates with HbF levels in a large cohort of sickle cell patients [43], this indicates that BCL11A variants, by modulating HbF levels, act as an important ameliorating factor of the SCA and it is likely they could help ameliorate other hemoglobin disorders. Genotyping of two other SNPs rs4671393 and rs7557939 in the Brazil Sickle cell disease cohorts have shown that these SNPs were more strongly associated with HbF level variation than rs11886868 [44].

In a recent study, we evaluated the association of rs11886868 of the BCL11A gene with mild, moderate, and severe groups of β-thalassemia and SCA. A significant association of CC genotype and C allele was observed with milder disease phenotype in β-thalassemia as well as SCA [45].

- Friend of Protein (FOP)

Friend of protein arginine methyltransferase I (FOP) has been reported to be one of the targets of protein arginine methyltransferase 1 (PRMT1), which stably interacts with chromatin [46]. Initially this protein was studied for its role in estrogen-dependent gene activation and in hemoglobin switching [46]. Studies have shown that knockdown of FOP in murine fetal liver cells transgenic for the β-globin locus significantly increased expression of both the mouse embryonic and human adult peripheral blood erythroid progenitors resulting in up-regulation of γ-globe and increased production of HbF [46]. As a result of this, HbF levels were reported to increase from background levels of 6% to 7% to an average of approximately 27%. It was observed that BCL11A levels were not altered interestingly, but levels of Sex determining region Y-box 6 (SOX6) protein appeared to be reduced. Therefore, there is a possibility that FOP depletion increases globin expression via reduction of SOX6.

- Sex determining region X-box 6 (SOX6 -SRY)

SOX6 plays an important role in the silencing of the embryonic globin genes. This gene encodes a member of the D subfamily of sex determining region y-related transcription factors. It is characterized by a conserved DNA-binding domain termed the high mobility group box and has the ability to bind the minor groove of DNA. The encoded protein is a transcriptional activator which is required for normal development of the central nervous system, chondrogenesis, and maintenance of cardiac and skeletal muscle cells. This protein interacts with other family members to activate gene expression. Alternative splicing leads to multiple transcript variants. First of all, SOX6 was observed to play a role in the silencing of the mouse embryonic globin genes. It binds to the murine γ-globin promoter as observed by Chromatin immune-precipitation [47]. It was also found that SOX6 interacts with BCL11A, although SOX6 strongly binds the globin gene promoters suggesting that the SOX6-BCL11A protein-protein interaction may involve chromatin looping [48]. SOX6 binding to the γ-globin promoters requires BCL11A. Studies have shown that the knockdown of SOX6 in cultured, primary human erythroblasts led to a small up-regulation of HbF but when combined with BCL11A knock-down, further enhanced HbF production [48].

- KLF1

KLF1, known as Erythroid Kruppel-like factor, is a zinc finger protein which binds the CACCC of the adult globin gene in mice as well as humans [49–50]. This protein is important for its expression responsible for ablation in mice causing embryonic lethality due to severe anemia [51–52]. Studies have shown that both endogenous mouse embryonic and human fetal globin gene expression are not properly down-regulated in the *Eklf*$^{-/-}$ mice. The haemoglobin switching role of this protein was identified in further studies [53–54]. A GWAS scan followed by linkage analysis of a family including 27 members showed that 10 out of 27 members had Hereditary persistence of fetalhemoglobin phenotype. In this study, a nonsense mutation in KLF1 gene was identified, which ablated the DNA binding domain, resulting in haploinsufficiency in the heterozygous state [53]. The HbF levels were found to vary among individual family members, indicating the influence of other genetic and environmental factors. In addition to the binding globin gene promoter, normal KLF1 was reported to show strong binding to the BCL11A promoter, thereby activating its expression in cultured, primary adult human erythroblasts. KLF1 has been found to mediate its switching effects through a dual mechanism, acting both on the globin and BCL11A promoters. Zhou et al. also found that reduced, but not absent, KLF1 levels in genetically altered mice resulted in markedly decreased levels of BCL11A mRNA and protein [54]. The researchers found that there was a strong binding of KLF1 to the Bcl11A promoter. Further, mouse embryonic and human fetal globin transgene expressions were found to be highly increased in the setting of reduced KLF1. Similar to this, it was found that when KLF1 was knocked down in cultured adult human erythroblasts, γ-globin gene expression was up-regulated [54]. Therefore, both compelling evidence from genetic and functional data suggests that KLF1 has a significant role in the fetal to adult switch. However, a 2- to 3-fold elevated expression in adult versus fetal cells, which results in KLF1's preferential association with the β-promoter in the former and the γ-promoters in the latter, is still not clear.

- HBSL1-MYB DNA region

In a GWAS, designed to identify polymorphisms associated with the variability of HbF expression in nonanemic humans, variants in the intergenic region between the HBSL1 and MYB genes were identified [55]. Data suggests that the intergenic area is most highly associated with HbF expression and consists of properties of a regulatory element [56]. The linkage to an equilibrium block, which is most closely associated with HbF levels, is between the HBS1L and MYB genes, which are present on opposite DNA strands. Three hypersensitive sites have been found within that region. These sites have been recognized as the characteristic marks of active chromatin, including histone acetylation and RNA polymerase II binding in erythroid, but not in nonerythroid cells [56]. HBS1L is supposed to be a housekeeping gene because it is ubiquitously expressed. Whereas MYB has more of a restrictive pattern of expression and is crucial for erythroid development.

Studies have compared the expression profiles of 5 genes within this region, including MYB and HBS1L, in the erythroid cultures of 12 persons with elevated and 14 persons with normal HbF levels [57]. In this study, both MYB and HBS1L were down-regulated in persons with elevated HbF levels, whereas the other 3 genes did not change in their level of expression. Overexpression of MYB inhibited-globin gene expression in human erythroleukemia cells, whereas overexpression of HBS1L was reported with no effect. The researchers speculated that low levels of MYB result in fewer cell-cycle events early in erythropoiesis and that early maturation of erythroblasts yields red cells containing higher levels of HbF [57]. Overall, MYB has a critical role in erythropoiesis, and studies suggest that it acts, in part, by transactivation of KLF1 and LMO2 expression. 84 studies involving genotyping and resequencing have found that rare missense mutations might provide further evidence for the involvement of MYB in modulating HbF levels [50].

- TR2/TR4 DR erythroid-definitive complex

A repressor of the human embryonic ε-globin gene, the direct repeat (DR) erythroid-definitive complex consists of a heterodimer of 2 orphan nuclear receptors, TR2 and TR4 [58–59]. In vitro studies have found that this dimer, along with the nuclear factor COUP TFII binds DRs in the ε-globin gene promoter. Later, it binds to a similar repeat with the γ-globin gene promoters [60]. Endogenous murine embryonic to adult globin gene and fetal to adult human γ-globin transgene switching is delayed in mice which are null for TR2/TR4. In contrast to this, enforced expression of a dominant negative TR4 results in both loss of endogenous embryonic gene expression and human γ-globin transgene silencing. A mutation at -117 of the γ-globin promoter was indicated to be associated with HPFH, thereby affecting a DR element and influencing factor binding, adding to the evidence that this heterodimer plays a role in stage-selective repression of the human γ-globin gene [61–62].

- COUP-TFII

COUP-TFII was known as one of the 2 factors required for transcription of the chicken ovalbumin gene [63]. COUP-TFII was later found to bind to the γ-globin promoter DR in vitro as well [64]. Mutation of DR elements resulted in derepression of γ-globin transgene expression in adult mice, indicating that DR sites are involved in fetal globin gene silencing. An in vitro model of primary human erythroblast development was used to show that the cytokine stem cell factor, through activation of the Erk1/2 and/or p38 mitogen activated protein kinase pathways, suppresses COUP-TFII expression at the mRNA and protein level, resulting in a large reduction in its binding to the γ-globin promoter.

- NF-E4

NF-E4 was identified as a component of the "stage selector protein," which binds to the stage selector element in the proximal-globin promoter in human K562 erythroleukemia cells; NF-E4, in conjunction with the ubiquitous transcription factor CP2, facilitates transcription of the γ-globin gene [65–66]. The stage selector element is conserved in species having γ-globin genes and is not present in species lacking HbF. The p22 NF-E4 acts as an "activator" of γ-globin transcription via interacting with CP2 to recruit p45 NF-E2 and subsequently RNA polymerase II to the promoter. Further evidence supporting a role for NFE4 in HbF production is that, an HPFH mutation at -202 creates a new binding site for the NF-E4-CP2 complex [67]. This alternate form, p14 NF-E4, apparently generated by translational initiation from an internal methionine, has been suggested to play a role in γ-globin gene down-regulation or silencing. The smaller isoform is abundant in adult erythroid cells, and although it did not bind the-globin promoter, it appears to interact with CP2 and might function to sequester NF-E2, which prevents complexing of activating factors at the γ-globin promoter. Enforced expression of p22 NF-E4 in transgenic mice harboring the human β-globin locus delayed the switch, without elevating the expression of HbF in the adult [67].

- GATA-1

GATA-1 is a member of zinc finger transcription factor and plays a seminal role in the development and differentiation of many cell types, including mega karyocytes, erythrocytes, eosinophils, and mast cells [68–69]. β-globin locus transcriptional activation can be resolved into discrete molecular steps involving the formation of distinct GATA-1 cofactor assemblies at the promoters and the Locus control region (LCR) [70]. Data suggest that GATA-1 can act both as a repressor and activator of gene transcription. Interaction between GATA-1 and the YY1 protein is involved in the silencing of the ε-globin gene in primate and non-primate species [71]. Moreover, binding of a GATA-1–FOG-1–NuRD complex was indicated to silence hematopoietic genes in erythroid cells [69, 72].

GATA-1 has multiple partners of proteins, including Stat3, Stat5, FOG-1, TAL-1, and Gfi-1b among others [73–75]. GATA-1 was firstly identified as a transactivator [73], however, its ability to mediate gene repression can be achieved through different DNA binding sequences, e.g. palindromic GATA-1 motifs and double GATA sites [76–77]. GATA-1 repressor activity has been implicated in naturally occurring mutations in the γ-globin genes which are associated with the persistent HbF synthesis after birth. These include point mutations at base -175 (T → C) and -173 (T → C) of the γ-globin promoter, which reduces GATA-1 binding and produces elevated HbF levels in humans and transgenic mice respectively [78]. Likewise, the -567 and -566 GATA-1 sites in the Gγ- and Aγ-globin promoter, respectively, have been found to be associated with gene silencing [79–80]. Amrolia et al. defined a repressor element in the γ-globin 5′-UTR, which was bound by a complex of two proteins, identified as GATA-1 and a ubiquitous negative regulator [81]. In a study, it was suggested that Stat3 binds the γ-globin 5′UTR to silence γ-globin transcription while GATA-1 binds the same region to enhance γ-promoter activity. Collectively, these studies suggest a model whereby GATA-1 acts as either a direct repressor or interacts with factors that bind nearby canonical sites to silence gene expression as proposed by Amrolia and co-workers [81].

In support for data provided by Harju-baker et al., a T3G mutation in the 567 GATA site of the gamma-globin gene in an Iranian-American family was reported to be associated with an HPFH phenotype by David Chui [80].

5.3. Induction of γ-globin gene expression

High HbF levels modulate the phenotype of the disease and ameloriate the severity of β-thalassemia and related complications led to an idea that reactivation of γ-globin gene will be a promising approach for the treatment of the disease [82–83]. Treatment strategies can be based on the following factors: an understanding pathophysiology of the disease; perspective of HbF to alter its manifestation; and that the developmental changes in γ-globin gene can be reversed by controling cellular and molecular regulatory mechanism [21]. Different classes of HbF inducers for clinical use have been reported.

Studies have shown that there are a number of inducers of the gamma-globin gene, like epigenetic modifiers of HbF and HbF inducers from the natural world.

- Epigenetic modifiers

If the molecular events occurring during haemoglobin switching are better understood, HbF expression could be more fully reactivated in adult cells and might lead to a cure for β-thalassemia.

The expression of human β-like globin genes are tissue- and developmental stage-specific in vivo. The mechanisms involved in the regulation of globin gene expression have been the subject of consideration for many years. Studies have led to the identification of cis- and trans-acting factors that regulate the expression of the β-globin gene cluster. Such studies also led to the recognition of the important role of epigenetic modifiers of globin gene expression. DNA methylation and histone acetylation are two of the most important epigenetic modifications that are involved in the regulation of most of the eukaryotic genes, including the genes of the globin family. Thus, targeting epigenetic silencing of the fetal globin genes can be a novel therapeutic approach for patients with β-thalassemia.

Epigenetic modifiers of HbF can be grouped in several classes, with different mechanisms of action. Different epigenetic modifiers of γ-globin gene are namely: erythropoietin, short chain fatty acids and cytotoxic agents, azacytidine, and hydroxycarbamide [84] (Table 1).

Many inducers inhibit histone deacethylase (HDAC) activity [85]. While most of the inducers exhibit inhibitory effects on cell growth, very few of them trigger increased γ-globin expression without effecting cell proliferation [86]. Erythroid precursor cells from β-thalassemia patients may differ in their response to the same inducer. Combined use of HbF inducers exhibiting different mechanism of action might improve the results.

- Cytotoxic agents

Observations that the use of cytotoxic agents helps to reactivate HbF synthesis during recovery from bone marrow suppression haves given hope on the possible use of cytotoxic agents for the treatment of serious haemoglobin disorders. Several cytotoxic agents that modify the pattern of erythropoiesis, increasing the expression of fetal (γ)-globin genes, have been explored over the past two decades [87–88]. Cytotoxic compounds put an end to actively cycling progenitors and control cellular growth to trigger rapid erythroid-regeneration and the formation of F cells. Cytotoxic drugs such as vinblastine [89], busulfan [90], cytosine arabinoside [91], and hydroxyurea [92–94] are known inducers of HbF in humans through this mechanism. Rapid regeneration of erythroid cells allows progenitors with an active eHbF program to be selectively recruited for maturation.

- Short-chain fatty acids (SCFAs)

Two different studies have reported that the infants of diabetic mothers have a delayed fetal-to-adult hemoglobin switch [95–96], while the exact underlying mechanisms are not clear, it is known that hydroxybutyrate is elevated during pregnancy induced diabeties in women. Perrine and colleagues observed that butyrate or other similar short chain fatty acids may act as effective inducers of fetal hemoglobin in sheep [95].

In support to the above observation, many other studies have shown that Sodium phenylbutyrate and arginine butyrate enhance both fetal and total hemoglobin levels in patients with sickle cell disease and beta thalassemia [97–106]. However, these SCFA derivatives also inhibit histone deacetylases, which generally inhibit erythroid cell proliferation. Therefore, these are not preferred as oral therapeutics that induce fetal (γ)-globin gene expression in beta hemoglobinopathies.

Loss of response to butyrates in long term therapy is observed which may be the result of antiproliferative effects on the bone marrow [107]. Two cohort studies have examined the efficacy of the oral butyrate derivative isobutyramide to induce HbF. In some studies no change in globin chain imbalance or in markers of ineffective erythropoiesis was noted, while in other study a drop in plasma free hemoglobin was observed. It has been suggested that the loss of response to long term butyrate therapy in patients with β-thalassemia may be because of the effects of these agents on other globin chains. It was shown that butyrate increases α-globin expression in progenitor-derived erythroid cells from patients with β-thalassemia. Thus, suggesting that the complementary effects of the butyrate-induced γ-globin expression on α/

http://dx.doi.org/10.5772/61441

β-chain imbalance in β-thalassemia may be decreased as a result of the associated increase in α-globin expression [108].

Using insilico modeling, Perrine and associates have tested several SCFA derivatives to deduce the functional group(s) required for γ-globin reactivation [109]. Compounds such as phenoxyacetic acid, and 2, 2 dimethylbutyric acid and α-methyl hydrocinnamic acid, induce Stat-5 cell signaling and the growth-related immediate early genes c-myc and cmyb to achieve HbF induction independent of HDAC inhibition; butyrate has similar effects [101,110].

Short chain fatty acids, like Phenylbutyrate and Valproic acid, are also known to induce HbF levels in vivo [111–112]. Animal model studies have shown that propionate, phenyl acetic, and phenylalkyl acids induces HbF in baboons, transgenic mice, cultures, and in primates [103, 113–115].

- DNA methyl transferase (DNMT) inhibitors

DNA methylation is an epigenetic method of modulating gene expression carried out by enzyme DNA methyltransferases (DNMT) in both eukaryotes and prokaryotes [116]. These enzymes catalyze the addition of a methyl group from a donor S-adenosylmethionine to the 5′ position of cytosine, predominantly within the CpG dinucleotide [117–118].

CpG methylation in the promoter of adult erythroid cells is known to silence γ-globin gene expression [119]. The cytosine analogues such as, 5-azacytidine and 5-aza-2′-deoxycytidine (decitabine), are known to inhibit DNMTs and can be used to reactivate γ-gene expression [120–122].

The γ-globin genes are structurally and functionally similar in baboons and humans and are developmentally silenced by methylation of CpG residues [123]. 5-Azacytidine was shown to increase HbF levels in baboons and sickle cell patients, but concerns over the carcinogenic effect of 5-azacytidine hampered its development for human treatment [124–126].

Another DNA methylation inhibitor adenosine-2 3-dialdehyde (Adox) is known to inhibit both DNA methylation and protein methylation including histone tail methylation. It is known to inhibit adenosylhomocysteine hydrolase activity, thereby indirectly inhibiting methyltransferases that catalyze adenosylmethionine to adenosylhomocysteine [127]. In order to test the effect of Adox to induce γ-globin, He et al. performed a series of studies. Firstly, they treated K562 cells and showed a dose response effect on activation. Next, they performed a time-course analysis of γ-globin induction by Adox. They observed that from day two, γ-globin expression was readily detected, but after day six, induction stopped suggesting that Adox could induce γ-globin very quick and it could also be metabolized during cell proliferation. Adox also induced a dose-dependent inhibition of in vitro proliferation of K562 cells. They also performed bisulfite DNA sequencing experiments on globin genes. Using decitabine as a positive control, they found that Adox significantly reduced DNA methylation. Together, these results suggested that Adox was a potent inducer of γ-globin expression in K562 cells [128].

In their previous study, the levels of histone mark H4R3me2s on the γ-globin promoter triggered by PRMT5 were significantly reduced in Adox-treated and decitabine-treated cells compared to untreated cells. PRMT5 inhibition by Adox treatment followed a dose response that occurred over the same drug concentration range as γ-globin induction, indicating specificity of Adox for γ-globin gene.

However, DNA hypomethylation by Adox treatment may not be a major cause of the reactivation γ-globin expression in human β-thalassemia cells. But we can't exclude the possibility that by Adox treatment, different erythroid specific transcription factors play roles upon γ-globin induction. Alternatively, histone modification or repressor complex (e.g., NURD complex) reconstitution might also contribute to the γ-globin gene reactivation [129–131].

- Histone Deacetylase (HDAC) inhibitors

Histone deacetylases (HDACs) remove the acetyl group from histones resulting in the formation of tightly supercoiled, transcriptionally silent, "heterochromatin" structure that exerts antagonistic epigenetic controls on gene expression through chromatin re-modeling resulting in gene activation or repression [132–136]. HDACs are also known to deacetylase non-histone proteins, including many regulatory genes and transcriptional factors involved in cell signalling path and metabolism [137–138]. These observations suggest that HDACs plays an important role as co-repressors and co-activators of gene expression [139].

Till now, 18 mammalian HDAC genes have been identified that have been classified into four groups based on sequence homologies and catalytic mechanism [138, 140]. Class I includes HDACs 1-3, 8 and are expressed ubiquitously and consist mainly of a deacetylase domain. Class II includes HDACs 4-7 and 9-10, and are highly expressed in muscle, brain, and T cells [141]. Class I, II, and IV HDACs are evolutionarily related Zn^{+}-dependent hydrolases whereas, Class III HDACs have homology with yeast HDAC, silent information regulator 2, and use nicotinamide adenine dinucleotide as a co-substrate [142]. They have an extended N-terminus, which serves as a target for post-translational modifications and protein-protein interactions, such as phosphorylation, important for their function and governing nuclear-cytoplasmic shuttling [143].

A study by Forsberg et al. have shown that some specific histone acetylation patterns play a role in β-globin switch in murines, suggesting that the HDACs might participate in a complex mechanism of γ-globin repression, hence can be used for pharmacological reactivation of γ-globin expression [85, 144].

Shalini et al. (2010) screened Class II HDAC family members. They choose this class because they are highly tissue-specific in expression and have nuclear localization and import signals required for cell proliferation and differentiation [145–147]. Histone deacetylase inhibitors, including sodium butyrate (NaB) and trichostatin A (TSA) and hemin are known to significantly alter the mRNA levels of HDAC7, -9, and -10 and histone deacetylase-related protein (HDRP) at the same time activating γ-globin expression, as the result of loss in HDAC activity at the promoter or can also be because of changes in the expression of other genes [147]. This was verified by studying siHDAC9 in K562 cells, a dose-dependent decrease in γ-globin gene expression was observed, where forced expression of HDAC9 reactivated the γ-globin expression [147]. This study suggests that HDAC9 might have a positive role in regulating γ-globin expression.

http://dx.doi.org/10.5772/61441

A rapid and efficient method for detecting HbF inducers, based on a recombinant DNA construct was developed by Skarpidi and colleagues [148]. In this method, the coding sequences of the firefly and renilla luciferase genes were substituted for the human γ-globin and β-globin genes, respectively. Many new HDAC inhibitors were identified in this system and were further confirmed in human erythroid progenitor cultures [148]. With the help of the same reporter system, Makala and Pace found a stable reporter system in human KU812 cells [149]. The chemical analogues of HDAC inhibitor FK228 were identified as novel HbF inducers in primary erythroid progenitors. Last two decades has seen tremendous growth to identify other agents, systems with the help of high throughput screening techniques. Using this approach, selective HDAC 1/2 inhibitors (e.g., ACY-957) which induced HbF were reported [150]. Studies with ACY-957 have demonstrated elevated HbF expression in human erythroid progenitors [151].

Inducer	Mechanism of action	References (a)
Peptiole nucleic acids (PNAs)	Artificial promoters	Wang et al. (1999)
Cisplatin and analogues	DNA-binding drug	Bianchi et al. (2000)
Triple-helix oligodeoxynucleotides	Activation of γ-globin gene promote	Xu et al. (2000)
Trichostatin	HDAC inhibitors	Marianna et al. (2001)
Tallimustine and analogues	DNA-binding drug	Bianchi et al. (2001)
Angelicin	DNA-binding drug	Lampronti et al. (2003)
Mithramycin	DNA-binding drug	Fibach et al. (2003)
Citarabine	Hypomethylation of DNA	Sauthararajah et al, 2003
Hydroxyurea	Inhibition of DNA synthesis	Fibach et al. (2003)
Apicidin	HDAC inhibitors	Witt et al. (2003)
Rapamycin	FRAP-mTOR signal transduction	Mischiati et al. (2003) Fibach et al. (2006)
Scriptaid	HDAC inhibitors	Johnson et al. (2005)

Table 1. Inducers of Fetal Hemoglobin in Erythroid Precursor Cells from Human Donors

5.4. Other novel agents under development

Usually, developing a novel agent from bench to bedside takes more than 20 years on an average; thus, repurposing that FDA approved agents is a strategy encouraged by drug companies and government funding agents to expand the agents available to treat β-hemoglobinopathies. One such agent is the FDA approved Tecfidera (dimethyl fumarate), used for the treatment of multiple sclerosis. This agent acts via mediating immunemodulatory actions [152] with limited side effects. Dimethyl fumarate activates NRF2 signaling involved in drug mediated HbF induction [153–154]. Researchers have reported that dimethyl fumarate induces γ-globin expression in KU812 and primary erythroid cells generated from sickle cell patients, thereby supporting repurposing of Tecfidera for SCD [155].

Another FDA approved agent pomalidomide is under development for SCD. This agent stimulates proliferation of erythroid progenitors and HbF induction [156]. In a pre-clinical study, pomalidomide was investigated in the SCD knockout transgenic mouse produced by Townes and colleagues and was shown to induce HbF similar to hydroxylurea without myelo suppression. This study led to a Phase 1 clinical trial completion [157–159].

Preclinical studies to support the repurpose of the monoamine oxidase inhibitor tranylcypromine for SCD have been completed. The nuclear receptors TR2 and TR4 repress γ-globin expression by association with the co-repressors DNMT1 and lysine-specific demethylase 1 (LSD1) [58–59]. LSD1 removes methyl groups from mono- and dimethyl histone H3 lysine 4 producing an activating epigenetic signature [160]. The role of LSD1 in globin gene regulation in human erythroid cells was examined by Shi and colleagues [161]. They demonstrated that LSD1 was inhibited by tranylcypromine which mediated and enhanced HbF expression. Subsequent pre-clinical studies using β-YAC transgenic mice treated with tranylcypromine produced HbF induction. This served the basis for a clinical trial to test the ability of this agent in order to induce HbF in β-hemoglobinopathy patients [16].

5.5. Clinical development of HbF inducer

Till date, the most successful HbF inducer in the pharmacological armamentarium of drugs is Hydroxurea (HU). The first description of HU treatment in patients with SCD dates back to the year 1984 [162]. Since then, HU was found to elevate HbF levels and decrease the clinical complications of SCD and finally in 1998 it became the only FDA approved drug for SCD. In a Multicenter Study of Hydroxyurea (MSH), adult subjects with SCD were randomized on HU therapy or placebo and individuals in the HU group had ~50% reduction in vaso-occlusive rates [163]. Patients with maximal change in HbF levels had the highest reduction in white blood cell counts, indicating a hematologic response was associated with the clinical response [164]. The MSH data also demonstrated that treatment with HU was not associated with significant toxicities and was effective at reducing healthcare costs associated with complications due to SCD [163, 165]. Long-term follow up of MSH patients up to 17.5 years reported that there was a reduction in mortality [166]. Similar to these results, it was observed in the 17-year open label Laikon Study of HU in Sickle Cell Syndromes [167]; the probability of 10-year survival was 86% and 65% for HU and non-HU patients, respectively [167].

5.6. HU treatment in children

The efficacy and safety in adult trials was proved, and therefore the investigations of HU were undertaken in children. A pilot study of HU (HUSOFT) was conducted in 28 children with SCD where HU therapy was found to be feasible, well tolerated, and efficacious in young children. In addition, based on liver, spleen scans, HU could possibly delay functional asplenia [168]. Long-term follow-up data of patients in the HUSOFT extension study showed a reduction in acute SCD complications, improved splenic function, and improved growth rates in children taking HU therapy [169]. Based on these findings, BABY-HUG, a Phase III randomized controlled trial, was conducted in children with SCD (mean age 13.6 months) [170]. The primary endpoints of improved splenic function and renal glomerular filtration rates were not achieved. HU was effective at reducing the acute complications of SCD, such as pain episodes, dactylitis, acute chest syndrome, and red blood transfusions [170]. The researchers were interested to use HU to prevent the long-term organ damage of SCD or to avoid chronic transfusions for children with severe phenotypes. Evidence of organ protection from HU in the current literature led to investigations of HU in this setting [171–173]. The Stroke With Transfusions Changing to Hydroxyurea (SWiTCH) study was a Phase III multicentred randomized trial compared the HU or phlebotomy with transfusions and chelation for the prevention of secondary stroke and reduction of transfusion iron overload [174–175]. There were no subsequent strokes on the transfusions/chelation arm but (10%) on the HU/phlebotomy arm. No major difference in liver iron content was found between the groups; therefore, the study was closed early. The investigators confirmed that the transfusions and chelation remain the standard of management of children with SCD and stroke complicated by iron overload [174]. Moreover, the studies in children have yet to demonstrate a role of HU in the prevention or management of chronic complications.

5.7. Natural inducers

Recently, scientists have conducted many studies to identify the natural remedies that could possibly be applied for the treatment of β-thalassemia (Table 2) [176]. Several studies have found that the extracts from medicinal plants for biomedical purposes [177–186] including therapeutic strategies can be used for the treatment of a number of diseases.

In case of hemoglobinopathies, only a few examples are available. For instance, the extract of Aegle Marmelos containing bergatene was found to activate erythroid differentiation and HbF induction in human leukemic K562 cells [187–188]. Citropten and bergatene are the two active ingredients in bergamot juice. They are potent inducers of Erythroid cell differentiation, $^{G}\gamma$-globin gene expression and fetal hemoglobin synthesis in human erythroid cells. Thus, it is known as a possible therapeutic approach for both β-thalassemia and Sickle cell anemia [187].

Another example of HbF inducer from the natural world is Angelicin, which can be found in the fruit of *Angelica arcangelica*. There is evidence demonstrating that angelicin is a strong inducer of Erythroid cell differentiation, improvement of the HbF synthesis, and γ-globin mRNA accumulation of human leukemia K562 cells [84, 179]. Red wine, particularly the skin of black grapes, contains resveratrol which mimics the HbF-inducing activity of HU. Its role in increasing the γ-globin mRNA in human erythroid precursors has been confirmed [84]. Since β-thalassemia cells present a high level of oxidative stress resulting in short time survival of erythroid cells in β-thalassemia patients, resveratrol which exhibits both antioxidant activity and HbF inducing property can be a very good HbF inducer from the natural world [88].

Rapamycin, which is isolated from *Streptomyces hygroscopicus*, is a bacterial species found in soil of Easter Island has the capability of increasing HbF production in cultures of erythroid precursors from β-thalassemia patients without any cytotoxicity or growth-inhibitory effect. Apart from Rapamycin, Mithramycin is a DNA-binding drug that is easily isolated from Streptomyces has the potential to induce γ-globin mRNA accumulation and HbF production in erythroid cells from healthy subjects as well as β-thalassemia patients [189].

Inducer	Source	Biological effects	References
Bergaptene	*A. marmelos*	Erythroid differentiation of K562 cells	Lampronti et al. (2003)
Angelicin	*A. arcangelica*	HbF production	Lampronti et al. (2003)
Rapamycin	*S. hygroscopicus*	HbF production	Mischiati et al. (2004)
Resveratrol	Redwine, grape skin and darakchasava	HbF production	Rodrigue et al. (2001)
Mithramycn	*Streptomyces* species	HbF production	Bianchi et al. (1999)
YiSui ShengXue Granule		Erythroid survival, proliferation, and terminaldifferentiation of K562 cells and HbF production	Zhang and Wu (2008)
Cucurbitacn D	Ethanol extract of Fructus trichosanthis, which is the fruit of Trichosanthes kirilowii MAXIM	HbF production and Erythroid differentiation of K562cells	Liu et al. (2010); Li et al. (2011)
Terminalia catappa distilled water active fraction (TCDWF)	*Terminalia catappa leaves*	Erythropoiesis, cell proliferation, and transcription	Aimola et al. (2014)

Table 2. Inducers of HbF from natural sources

6. Discussion and conclusion

The Human Genome Project has improved efforts of developing gene-based therapy for β-hemoglobinopathies alongside chemical inducers. GWAS have found certain major genetic modifiers of γ-globin, including -158 XmnI HBG2, HBS1-MYB and BCL11A accounting for ~50% of inherited HbF variance [190–191]. Orkin and colleagues advanced the field significantly by defining mechanisms through which BCL11A repressed γ-globin expression and holds the promise for the development of gene-based therapy in the future.

The occurrence of inherited mutations in KLF1 that produce HPFH suggested that this factor is a viable target for gene therapy and might be accomplished by RNAi technology to create a haploinsufficiency state. Promising molecular targets such as KLF1 and BCL11A for therapeutic efforts aimed at HbF induction have been identified: however, additional pre-clinical data are needed before manipulation of transcription factors can be translated into therapeutic options at the bedside.

Agents which improve HbF synthesis represent a rational approach for the treatment of β-thalassemia. For more than three decades, many chemical agents have been tested in tissue culture as HbF inducers, but few have crossed the path from clinical trials and have reached to the bedside. One major roadblock is the lack of suitable pre-clinical models to test agents in vivo. Baboon studies led to the clinical development of HU, butyrate, decitabine, and

HQK-1001 in SCD and β-thalassemia [93, 120–121, 124–125, 192–197]. With the establishment of SCD mouse models, newer agents such as pomalidomide have been progressed to clinical trials, however, the limited availability of the knockout SCD mouse model has affected progress in this area [155]. Townes and colleagues had designed a second knockin SCD mouse model with γ-globin and β-globin constructs [157]. However, HbF induction has not been effectively achieved with HU therapy (Pace, unpublished data). Therefore, the knock-in mouse may not be ideal for future pre-clinical drug screens. An alternative model, the β-YAC mouse was used to confirm in vivo HbF induction by 5-azacytidine, scriptaid, and transcyclomide showing the utility of this mouse for pre-clinical drug screening [161, 198–199]. Currently, very few agents are in clinical trials targeting HbF induction and drugs aimed at other complications of SCD, such as nitric oxide deficiency, endothelium antagonist, anti-platelet agents, anti-sickle agents, and so forth are still under development (clinicaltrials.gov). These can be combined with HU or other HbF inducers to produce an additive or synergistic clinic benefit [155].

Despite the success of HU in clinical trials conducted on adults and children and its proven safety and efficacy, it remains underutilized in SCD [163–164, 166, 168–170, 173, 200–201]. Possible causes include: (1) limited access to comprehensive sickle cell medical care; 2) lack of coordination between subspecialists and community based clinicians; 3) concern over potential genotoxicity; and 4) lack of patient adherence with the medication regimen. Future studies are needed to address early initiation of HU, the role of HU therapy in prevention of chronic complications, and improved methods for HU therapy delivery to all patients with SCD. There remains a question about the optimal age to initiate HU therapy. The Baby HUG trial established safety in young children, but additional clinical safety data are needed for children <6 months at the highest risk of infection and spleen and kidney dysfunction. Whether the early HU therapy administration will prevent the γ- to β-globin switch has not been demonstrated.

Curative therapy for SCD and β-thalassemia includes hematopoietic stem cell transplantation, however, this option is limited by the availability of suitable donors in <20% of children with SCD [202–203]. Ongoing clinical trials exploring alternative approaches such as matched unrelated donors and the development of new regimens using haplo-identical donors in the future will increase the transplant option for the majority of SCD patients [204]. Another approach to cure β-hemoglobinopathies is efforts to develop gene therapy, e.g., recently there was a successful treatment of two β-thalassemia patients with a modified β-globin lentivirus based vector. This progress holds promise for SCD patients [205–206].

Landmark studies have developed an excitement that fully differentiated somatic cells can be reprogrammed to make induced pluripotent stem cells [207]. Subsequent studies demonstrated rectification of a mouse model of SCD using this innovative approach, therefore opened the way to the use of these cells to cure β-hemoglobinopathies beside few limitations [208]. One limitation was the inability to restore all hematopoietic lineages with induced pluripotent stem cells which precludes using human therapy [209]. Therefore, until transplantation and gene therapy is more widely available, chemical inducers of HbF remain the most effective way to treat β-thalassemia and SCD.

Author details

Anjana Munshi[1*], Sneha Dadeech[2], M. Sai Babu[2] and Preeti Khetarpal[1]

*Address all correspondence to: anjanadurani@yahoo.co.in

1 Centre for Human Genetics, Central University of Punjab, Bathinda, India

2 Department of Molecular Biology, Institute of Genetics and Hospital for Genetic Diseases, Osmania University, Hyderabad, India

References

[1] Galehdari H, Salehi B, Azmoun S, Keikhaei B, Zandian KM, Pedram M. Comprehensive spectrum of the β-Thalassemia mutations in Khuzestan, southwest Iran. Hemoglobin. 2010; 34(5):461-8.

[2] Kohne E. Hemoglobinopathies: clinical manifestations, diagnosis, and treatment. Dtsch Arztebl Int. 2011; 108(31-32):532-40.

[3] Trehan A, Sharma N, Das R, Bansal D, Marwaha RK. Clinicoinvestigational and demographic profile of children with thalassemia major. Indian J Hematol Blood Transfus. 2015; 31(1):121-6.

[4] Thein SL. Pathophysiology of beta thalassemia—a guide to molecular therapies. Hematology Am Soc Hematol Educ Program. 2005:31-7.

[5] Weatherall DJ. Phenotype-genotype relationships in monogenic disease: lessons from the thalassaemias. Nat Rev Genet. 2001; 2(4):245-55.

[6] Rund D, Rachmilewitz E. Beta-thalassemia. N Engl J Med. 2005; 353(11):1135-46.

[7] Cao A, Galanello R. Beta-thalassemia. Genet Med. 2010; 12(2):61-76.

[8] Thein SL. Genetic association studies in β-hemoglobinopathies. Hematology Am Soc Hematol Educ Program. 2013; 2013:354-61.

[9] Galanello R, Origa R. Beta-thalassemia. Orphanet J Rare Dis. 2010; 5:11.

[10] Cao A, Moi P, Galanello R. Recent advances in β-thalassemias. Pediatr Rep. 2011; 3(2):17.

[11] Nienhuis AW, Nathan DG. Pathophysiology and Clinical Manifestations of the β-Thalassemias. Cold Spring Harb Perspect Med. 2012; 2(12):011726.

[12] Olivieri NF, Pakbaz Z, Vichinsky E. Hb E/beta-thalassaemia: a common & clinically diverse disorder. Indian J Med Res. 2011; 134:522-31.

[13] Premawardhena A, De Silver S, Arambepola M, Olivieri NF, Vichinsky EP, Merson L, Muraco G, Allen A, Fisher C, Peto T, Weatherall DJ. Hemoglobin E-beta-thalassemia: Progress report from the International Study Group. Ann N Y Acad Sci. 2005; 1054:33-9.

[14] Joly P, Pondarre C, Badens C. Beta-thalassemias: molecular, epidemiological, diagnostical and clinical aspects. Ann Biol Clin (Paris). 2014; 72(6):639-668.

[15] Bard H, Prosmanne J. Relative rates of fetal hemoglobin and adult hemoglobin synthesis in cord blood of infants of insulin-dependent diabetic mothers. Pediatrics. 1985; 75(6): 1143-7.

[16] Bard H, Prosmanne J. Elevated levels of fetal hemoglobin synthesis in infants with bronchopulmonary dysplasia. Pediatrics. 1990; 86(2):193-6.

[17] Bard H, Lachance C, Widness JA, Gagnon C. The reactivation of fetal hemoglobin synthesis during anemia of prematurity. Pediatr Res. 1994; 36(2):253-6.

[18] Bard H, Gagnon C, Peri KG. HbF synthesis during stress erythropoiesis as determined by gamma-mRNA/non-alpha-mRNA quantification. Pediatr Res. 1999; 45(51):684-6.

[19] Bard H. The effect of placental insufficiency on fetal and adult hemoglobin synthesis. Am J Obstet Gynecol. 1974; 120(1):67-72.

[20] Blau CA. Therapy for globin-chain disorders. N Engl J Med. 1993; 329(5):364.

[21] Stamatoyannopoulos G, Nienhuis AW. Therapeutic approaches to hemoglobin switching in treatment of hemoglobinopathies. Annu Rev Med. 1992; 43:497-521.

[22] Karimi M, Haghpanah S, Taher AT, Cappellini MD. β-Thalassemia: New Therapeutic Modalities, Genetics, Complications, and Quality of Life. Anemia. 2012; 2012:902067.

[23] Breda L, Rivella S, Zuccato C, Gambari R. Combining gene therapy and fetal hemoglobin induction for treatment of β-thalassemia. Expert Rev Hematol. 2013; 6(3): 255-64.

[24] Fathallah H, Atweh GF. DNA hypomethylation therapy for hemoglobin disorders: molecular mechanisms and clinical applications. Blood Rev. 2006; 20(4):227-34.

[25] Ronzoni L, Sonzogni L, Fossati G, Modena D, Trombetta E, Porretti L, Cappellini MD. Modulation of gamma globin genes expression by histone deacetylase inhibitors: an in vitro study. Br J Haematol. 2014; 165(5):714-21.

[26] Mtatiro SN, Makani J, Mmbando B, Thein SL, Menzel S, Cox SE. Genetic variants at HbF-modifier loci moderate anemia and leukocytosis in sickle cell disease in Tanzania. Am J Hematol. 2015; 90(1):1-4.

[27] Svasti S, Paksua S, Nuchprayoon I, Winichagoon P, Fucharoen S. Characterization of a novel deletion causing (deltabeta)0-thalassemia in a Thai family. Am J Hematol. 2007; 82(2):155-61.

[28] Weatherall DJ. Phenotype-genotype relationships in monogenic disease: lessons from the thalassaemias. Nat Rev Genet. 2001; 2(4):245-55.

[29] Galanello R, Origa R. Beta-thalassemia. Orphanet J Rare Dis. 2010; 5:11.

[30] Nemati H, Rahimi Z, Bahrami G. The Xmn1 polymorphic site 5' to the (G)gamma gene and its correlation to the (G)gamma:(A)gamma ratio, age at first blood transfusion and clinical features in beta-thalassemia patients from Western Iran. Mol Biol Rep. 2010; 37(1):159-64.

[31] Pandey S, Pandey S, Mishra RM, Sharma M, Saxena R. Genotypic influence of α-deletions on the phenotype of Indian sickle cell anemia patients. Korean J Hematol. 2011; 46(3):192-5.

[32] Dadheech S, Jain S, Madhulatha D, Sharma V, Joseph J, Jyothy A, Munshi A. Association of Xmn1 -158 γG variant with severity and HbF levels in β-thalassemia major and sickle cell anaemia. Mol Biol Rep. 2014; 41(5):3331-7.

[33] Kawata H, Yamada K, Shou Z, Mizutani T, Yazawa T, Yoshino M, Sekiguchi T, Kajitani T, Miyamoto K. Zinc-fingers and homeoboxes (ZHX) 2, a novel member of the ZHX family, functions as a transcriptional repressor. Biochem J. 2003; 373(3):747-57.

[34] Spear BT, Jin L, Ramasamy S, Dobierzewska A. Transcriptional control in the mammalian liver: liver development, perinatal repression, and zonal gene regulation. Cell Mol Life Sci. 63(24):2922-38.

[35] de Andrade TG, Peterson KR, Cunha AF, Moreira LS, Fattori A, Saad ST, Costa FF. Identification of novel candidate genes for globin regulation in erythroid cells containing large deletions of the human beta-globin gene cluster. Blood Cells Mol Dis. 2006; 37(2):82-90.

[36] Perincheri S, Dingle RW, Peterson ML, Spear BT. Hereditary persistence of alpha-fetoprotein and H19 expression in liver of BALB/cJ mice is due to a retrovirus insertion in the Zhx2 gene. Proc Natl Acad Sci U S A. 2005; 102(2):396-401.

[37] Garner C, Silver N, Best S, Menzel S, Martin C, Spector TD, Thein SL. Quantitative trait locus on chromosome 8q influences the switch from fetal to adult hemoglobin. Blood. 2004; 104(7):2184-6.

[38] Aussara Panyaa, Nunghathai Sawasdeeb, Chatchawan Srisawata, Pa-thai Yenchitsomanusb, Chayanon Peerapittayamongkola. Expression of zinc finger and homeobox 2 in erythroleukaemic cells and gamma-globin expression. ScienceAsia. 2010; 36:342-345.

[39] De Andrade T, Moreira L, Duarte A, Lanaro C, De Albuquerque D, Saad S, Costa F. Expression of new red cell-related genes in erythroid differentiation. Biochem Genet. 2010; 48(1-2):164-71.

[40] Liu P, Keller JR, Ortiz M, Tessarollo L, Rachel RA, Nakamura T, Jenkins NA, Copeland NG. Bcl11a is essential for normal lymphoid development. Nat. Immunol. 2003; 4:525-532.

[41] Weniger MA, Pulford K, Gesk S, Ehrlich S, Banham AH, Lyne L, Martin-Subero JI, Siebert R, Dyer MJ, Möller P, Barth TF. Gains of the proto-oncogene BCL11A and nuclear accumulation of BCL11A(XL) protein are frequent in primary mediastinal B-cell lymphoma. Leukemia. 2006; 20(10):1880-2.

[42] Satterwhite E, Sonoki T, Willis TG, Harder L, Nowak R, Arriola EL, Liu H, Price HP, Gesk S, Steinemann D, Schlegelberger B, Oscier DG, Siebert R, Tucker PW, Dyer MJ. The BCL11 gene family: involvement of BCL11A in lymphoid malignancies. Blood. 2001; 98(12):3413-20.

[43] Uda M, Galanello R, Sanna S, Lettre G, Sankaran VG, Chen W, Usala G, Busonero F, Maschio A, Albai G, Piras MG, Sestu N, Lai S, Dei M, Mulas A, Crisponi L, Naitza S, Asunis I, Deiana M, Nagaraja R, Perseu L, Satta S, Cipollina MD, Sollaino C, Moi P, Hirschhorn JN, Orkin SH, Abecasis GR, Schlessinger D, Cao A. Genome-wide association study shows BCL11A associated with persistent fetal hemoglobin and amelioration of the phenotype of beta-thalassemia. Proc Natl Acad Sci U S A. 2008; 105(5): 1620-5.

[44] Lettre G, Sankaran VG, Bezerra MA, Araújo AS, Uda M, Sanna S, Cao A, Schlessinger D, Costa FF, Hirschhorn JN, Orkin SH. DNA polymorphisms at the BCL11A, HBS1L-MYB, and beta-globin loci associate with fetal hemoglobin levels and pain crises in sickle cell disease. Proc Natl Acad Sci U S A. 2008; 105(33):11869-74.

[45] SnehaDadheech, D. Madhulatha D, SumanJjain, James Joseph , A Jyothy, AnjanaMunshi. Association of BCL11A Genetic Variant (rs11886868) with severity in β-Thalassemia Major and Sickle Cell Anemia. Indian J Med Res (2015) (Accepted for publication in IJMR).

[46] van Dijk TB, Gillemans N, Pourfarzad F, van Lom K, von Lindern M, Grosveld F, Philipsen S. Fetal globin expression is regulated by Friend of Prmt1. Blood. 2010; 116(20):4349-52.

[47] Yi Z, Cohen-Barak O, Hagiwara N, Kingsley PD, Fuchs DA, Erickson DT, Epner EM, Palis J, Brilliant MH. Sox6 directly silences epsilon globin expression in definitive erythropoiesis. PLoS Genet. 2006; 2(2):14.

[48] Xu J, Sankaran VG, Ni M, Menne TF, Puram RV, Kim W, Orkin SH. Transcriptional silencing of gamma-globin by BCL11A involves long-range interactions and cooperation with SOX6. Genes Dev. 2010; 24(8):783-798.76.

[49] Miller IJ, Bieker JJ. A novel, erythroid cell-specific murine transcription factor that binds to the CACCC element and is related to the Kruppel family of nuclear proteins. Mol Cell Biol. 1993; 13(5):2776-2786.

[50] Donze D, Townes TM, Bieker JJ. Role of Erythroid Kruppel-like factor in huma gamma- to beta-globin gene switching. J Biol Chem. 1995; 270(4):1955-1959.

[51] Perkins AC, Sharpe AH, Orkin SH. Lethal betathalassaemia in mice lacking the Erythroid CACCC-transcription factor EKLF. Nature. 1995; 375(6529):318-322.

[52] Nuez B, Michalovich D, Bygrave A, Ploemacher R, Grosveld F. Defective haematopoiesis in fetal liver resulting from inactivation of the EKLF gene. Nature. 1995; 375(6529):316-318.

[53] Borg J, Papadopoulos P, Georgitsi M, Gutiérrez L, Grech G, Fanis P, Phylactides M, Verkerk AJ, van der Spek PJ, Scerri CA, Cassar W, Galdies R, van Ijcken W, Ozgür Z, Gillemans N, Hou J, Bugeja M, Grosveld FG, von Lindern M, Felice AE, Patrinos GP, Philipsen S. Haploinsufficiency for the erythroid transcription factor KLF1 causes hereditary persistence of fetal hemoglobin. Nat Genet. 2010; 42(9):801-805.

[54] Zhou D, Liu K, Sun CW, Pawlik KM, Townes TM. KLF1 regulates BCL11A expression and gamma- to beta-globin gene switching. Nat Genet. 2010; 42(9):742-744.

[55] Thein SL, Menzel S, Peng X, Best S, Jiang J, Close J, Silver N, Gerovasilli A, Ping C, Yamaguchi M, Wahlberg K, Ulug P, Spector TD, Garner C, Matsuda F, Farrall M, Lathrop M. Intergenic variants of HBS1L-MYB are responsible for a major quantitative trait locus on chromosome 6q23 influencing fetal hemoglobin levels in adults. Proc Natl Acad Sci U S A. 2007; 104(27):11346-11351.

[56] Wahlberg K, Jiang J, Rooks H, Jawaid K, Matsuda F, Yamaguchi M, Lathrop M, Thein SL, Best S. The HBS1LMYB intergenic interval associated with elevated HbF levels shows characteristics of a distal regulatory region in erythroid cells. Blood. 2009; 114(6):1254-1262.

[57] Jiang J, Best S, Menzel S, Silver N, Lai MI, Surdulescu GL, Spector TD, Thein SL. cMYB is involved in the regulation of fetal hemoglobin production in adults. Blood. 2006; 108(3):1077-1083.

[58] Tanabe O, Katsuoka F, Campbell AD, Song W, Yamamoto M, Tanimoto K, Engel JD. An embryonic/fetal beta-type globin gene repressor contains a nuclear receptor TR2/TR4 heterodimer. EMBO J. 2002; 21(13):3434-3442.

[59] Tanabe O, McPhee D, Kobayashi S, Shen Y, Brandt W, Jiang X, Campbell AD, Chen YT, Chang Cs, Yamamoto M, Tanimoto K, Engel JD. Embryonic and fetal beta-globin gene repression by the orphan nuclear receptors, TR2 and TR4.EMBO J. 2007; 26(9): 2295-2306.

[60] Omori A, Tanabe O, Engel JD, Fukamizu A, Tanimoto K. Adult stage gamma-globin silencing is mediated by a promoter direct repeat element. Mol Cell Biol. 2005; 25(9): 3443-3451.

[61] Berry M, Grosveld F, Dillon N. A single point mutation is the cause of the Greek form of hereditary persistence of fetal haemoglobin. Nature. 1992; 358(6386):499-502.

[62] Collins FS, Mentherall JE, Yamakawa M, Pan J, Weissman SM, Forget BG. A point mutation in the A gamma-globin gene promoter in Greek hereditary persistence of fetal haemoglobin. Nature. 1985; 313(6000):325-326.

[63] Sagami I, Tsai SY, Wang H, Tsai MJ, O'Malley BW. Identification of two factors required for transcription of the ovalbumin gene. Mol Cell Biol. 1986; 6(12):4259-4267.

[64] Filipe A, Li Q, Deveaux S, Godin I, Roméo PH, Stamatoyannopoulos G, Mignotte V. Regulation of embryonic/fetal globin genes by nuclear hormone receptors: A novel perspective on hemoglobin switching. EMBO J. 1999; 18(3):687-697.

[65] Jane SM, Nienhuis AW, Cunningham JM. Hemoglobin switching in man and chicken is mediated by a heteromeric complex between the ubiquitous transcription factor CP2 and a developmentally specific protein. EMBO J. 1995;14(1):97-105.

[66] Zhou W, Zhao Q, Sutton R, Cumming H, Wang X, Cerruti L, Hall M, Wu R, Cunningham JM, Jane SM. The role of p22 NF-E4 in human globin gene switching. J Biol Chem. 2004; 279(25):26227-32.

[67] Jane SM, Gumucio DL, Ney PA, Cunningham JM, Nienhuis AW. Methylation-enhanced binding of Sp1 to the stage selector element of the human gamma-globin gene promoter may regulate development specificity of expression. Mol Cell Biol. 1993; 13(6):3272-3281.

[68] Wilson NK, Foster SD, Wang X, Knezevic K, Schütte J, Kaimakis P, Chilarska PM, Kinston S, Ouwehand WH, Dzierzak E, Pimanda JE, de Bruijn MF, Göttgens B. Combinatorial transcriptional control in blood stem/progenitor cells: genome-wide analysis of ten major transcriptional regulators. Cell Stem Cell. 2010; 7(4):532-44.

[69] Chakalova L, Fraser P. Organization of transcription. Cold Spring Harb Perspect Biol. 2010; 2(9):000729.

[70] Kollias G, Wrighton N, Hurst J, Grosveld F. Regulated expression of human A gamma-, beta-, and hybrid gamma beta-globin genes in transgenic mice: manipulation of the developmental expression patterns. Cell. 1986; 46(1):89-94.

[71] Dzierzak E. Opening act in a hematopoietic program. Blood. 2009; 114(2):229-230.

[72] Magram J, Chada K, Costantini F. Developmental regulation of a cloned adult beta-globin gene in transgenic mice. Nature. 1985; 315(6017):338-340.

[73] Cantor AB1, Orkin SH. Transcriptional regulation of erythropoiesis: an affair involving multiple partners. Oncogene. 2002; 21(21):3368-76.

[74] Ezoe S, Matsumura I, Gale K, Satoh Y, Ishikawa J, Mizuki M, Takahashi S, Minegishi N, Nakajima K, Yamamoto M, Enver T, Kanakura Y. GATA transcription factors inhibit cytokine-dependent growth and survival of a hematopoietic cell line through the inhibition of STAT3 activity. J Biol Chem. 2005; 280(13):13163-70.

[75] Grosveld F1, Rodriguez P, Meier N, Krpic S, Pourfarzad F, Papadopoulos P, Kolodziej K, Patrinos GP, Hostert A, Strouboulis J. Isolation and characterization of hema-

topoietic transcription factor complexes by in vivo biotinylation tagging and mass spectrometry. Ann N Y Acad Sci. 2005; 1054:55-67.

[76] Trainor CD, Omichinski JG, Vandergon TL, Gronenborn AM, Clore GM, Felsenfeld G. A palindromic regulatory site within vertebrate GATA-1 promoters requires both zinc fingers of the GATA-1 DNA-binding domain for high-affinity interaction. Mol Cell Biol. 1996; 16:2238-2247.

[77] Trainor CD, Ghirlando R, Simpson MA. GATA zinc finger interactions modulate DNA binding and transactivation. J Biol Chem. 2000; 275:28157-28166.

[78] Magis W, Martin DI. HMG-I binds to GATA motifs: implications for an HPFH syndrome. Biochem Biophys Res Commun. 1995; 214:927-933.

[79] Chen Z, Luo HY, Basran RK, Hsu TH, Mang DW, Nuntakarn L, Rosenfield CG, Patrinos GP, Hardison RC, Steinberg MH, Chui DH. A T-to-G transversion at nucleotide -567 upstream of HBG2 in a GATA-1 binding motif is associated with elevated hemoglobin F. Mol Cell Biol. 2008; 28(13):4386-93.

[80] Harju-Baker S, Costa FC, Fedosyuk H, Neades R, Peterson KR. Silencing of Agamma-globin gene expression during adult definitive erythropoiesis mediated by GATA-1-FOG-1-Mi2 complex binding at the -566 GATA site. Mol Cell Biol. 2008; 28(10): 3101-13.

[81] Amrolia PJ, Cunningham JM, Ney P, Nienhuis AW, Jane SM. Identification of two novel regulatory elements within the 5'-untranslated region of the human A gamma-globin gene. J Biol Chem. 1995; 270(21):12892-8.

[82] Haley JD, Smith DE, Schwedes J, Brennan R, Pearce C, Moore C, Wang F, Petti F, Grosveld F, Jane SM, Noguchi CT, Schechter AN. Identification and characterization of mechanistically distinct inducers of gamma-globin transcription. Biochem Pharmacol. 2003; 66(9):1755-68.

[83] Mabaera R, Greene MR, Richardson CA, Conine SJ, Kozul CD, Lowrey CH. Neither DNA hypomethylation nor changes in the kinetics of erythroid differentiation explain 5-azacytidine's ability to induce human fetal hemoglobin. Blood. 2008; 111(1): 411-20.

[84] El-Beshlawy A, Hamdy M, El Ghamrawy M. Fetal globin induction in beta-thalassemia. Hemoglobin. 2009; 33(1):197-203.

[85] Cao H. Pharmacological induction of fetal hemoglobin synthesis using histone deacetylase inhibitors. Hematology. 2004; 9:223-233.

[86] Gambari R, Fibach E. Medicinal chemistry of fetal hemoglobin inducers for treatment of beta-thalassemia. Curr Med Chem. 2007; 14(2):199-212.

[87] Fathallah H, Atweh GF. Induction of fetal hemoglobin in the treatment of sickle cell disease. Hematology Am Soc Hematol Educ Program. 2006:58-62.

[88] Gambari R, Fibach E. Medicinal chemistry of fetal hemoglobin inducers for treatment of beta-thalassemia. Curr Med Chem. 2007; 14(2):199-212.

[89] Veith R, Galanello R, Papayannopoulou T, Stamatoyannopoulos G. Stimulation of f-cell production in patients with sickle-cell anemia treated with cytarabine or hydroxyurea. N Engl J Med. 1985; 313(25):1571-5.

[90] Liu DP, Liang CC, Ao ZH, Jia PC, Chen SS, Wang RX, et al. Treatment of severe beta-thalassemia (patients) with myleran. Am J Hematol. 1990; 33:50-55.

[91] Papayannopoulou T, Torrealba de Ron A, Veith R, Knitter G, Stamatoyannopoulos G. Arabinosylcytosine induces fetal hemoglobin in baboons by perturbing erythroid cell differentiation kinetics. Science. 1984; 224:617-619.

[92] Galanello R, Stamatoyannopoulos G, Papayannopoulou T. Mechanism of Hb F stimulation by S-stage compounds. In vitro studies with bone marrow cells exposed to 5-azacytidine, are-C, or hydroxyurea. J Clin Invest. 1988; 81:1209-1216.

[93] Musallam KM, Taher AT, Cappellini MD, Sankaran VG. Clinical experience with fetal hemoglobin induction therapy in patients with β-thalassemia. Blood. 2013; 121(12):2199-212; quiz 2372.

[94] Bayanzay K, Khan R. Meta-analysis on effectiveness of hydroxyurea to treat transfusion-dependent beta-thalassemia. Hematology. 2014 Dec 23. [Epub ahead of print].

[95] Perrine SP, Greene MF, Faller DV. Delay in the fetal globin switch in infants of diabetic mothers. N Engl J Med. 1985; 312(6):334-8.

[96] Bard H, Prosmanne J. Relative rates of fetal hemoglobin and adult hemoglobin synthesis in cord blood of infants of insulin-dependent diabetic mothers. Pediatrics. 1985; 75(6):1143-7.

[97] Perrine SP, Ginder GD, Faller DV, Dover GH, Ikuta T, Witkowska HE, Cai SP, Vichinsky EP, Olivieri NF. A short-term trial of butyrate to stimulate fetal-globin-gene expression in the beta-globin disorders. N Engl J Med. 1993; 328(2):81-6.

[98] Little JA, Dempsey NJ, Tuchman M, Ginder GD. Metabolic persistence of fetal hemoglobin. Blood. 1995; 85:1712-8.

[99] Atweh GF, Sutton M, Nassif I, Boosalis V, Dover GJ, Wallenstein S, Wright E, McMahon L, Stamatoyannopoulos G, Faller DV, Perrine SP. Sustained induction of fetal hemoglobin by pulse butyrate therapy in sickle cell disease. Blood. 1999; 93(6):1790-7.

[100] Steinberg MH, Rodgers GP. Pathophysiology of sickle cell disease: role of cellular and genetic modifiers. Semin Hematol. 2001; 38(4):299-306.

[101] Boosalis MS, Bandyopadhyay R, Bresnick EH, Pace BS, Van DeMark K, Zhang B, Faller DV, Perrine SP. Short-chain fatty acid derivatives stimulate cell proliferation and induce STAT-5 activation. Blood. 2001; 97(10):3259-67.

[102] Pace BS, White GL, Dover GJ, Boosalis MS, Faller DV, Perrine SP. Short-chain fatty acid derivatives induce fetal globin expression and erythropoiesis in vivo. Blood. 2002; 100:4640-4648.

[103] Perrine SP. Fetal globin induction—can it cure beta thalassemia? Hematology Am Soc Hematol Educ Program. 2005:38-44.

[104] Perrine SP, Castaneda SA, Boosalis MS, White GL, Jones BM, Bohacek R. Induction of fetal globin in beta-thalassemia: Cellular obstacles and molecular progress. Ann N Y Acad Sci. 2005; 1054:257-65.

[105] Castaneda S, Boosalis MS, Emery D, Thies A, Faller DV, Perrine SP. Enhancement of growth and survival and alterations in Bcl-family proteins in beta-thalassemic erythroid progenitors by novel short-chain fatty acid derivatives. Blood Cells Mol Dis. 2005; 35(2):217-26.

[106] Perrine SP. Fetal globin stimulant therapies in the beta-hemoglobinopathies: principles and current potential. Pediatr Ann. 2008; 37(5):339-46.

[107] Atweh GF, Sutton M, Nassif I, Boosalis V, Dover GJ, Wallenstein S, Wright E, McMahon L, Stamatoyannopoulos G, Faller DV, Perrine SP. Sustained induction of fetal hemoglobin by pulse butyrate therapy in sickle cell disease. Blood. 1999; 93(6):1790-7.

[108] Fathallah H, Taher A, Bazarbachi A, Atweh GF. Differences in response to fetal hemoglobin induction therapy in beta-thalassemia and sickle cell disease. Blood Cells Mol Dis. 2009; 43(1):58-62.

[109] Boosalis MS, Ikuta T, Pace BS, da Fonseca S, White GL, Faller DV, Perrine SP. Abrogation of IL-3 requirements and stimulation of hematopoietic cell proliferation in vitro and in vivo by carboxylic acids. Blood Cells Mol Dis. 1997; 23(3):434-42.

[110] Kutlar A, Meiler S, Swerdlow P, Knight R. Thalidomide and its analogs for hemoglobinopathies: two birds with one stone? Expert Rev Hematol. 2012; 5(1):9-11.

[111] Collins AF, Dover GJ, Luban NL. Increased fetal hemoglobin production in patients receiving valproic acid for epilepsy. Blood. 1994; 84:1690-1691.

[112] Dover GJ, Brusilow S, Charache S. Induction of fetal hemoglobin production in subjects with sickle cell anemia by oral sodium phenylbutyrate. Blood. 1994; 84(1): 339-43.

[113] Liakopoulou E, Blau CA, Li Q, Josephson B, Wolf JA, Fournarakis B, Raisys V, Dover G, Papayannopoulou T, Stamatoyannopoulos G. Stimulation of fetal hemoglobin production by short chain fatty acids. Blood. 1995; 86(8):3227-35.

[114] Torkelson S, White B, Faller DV, Phipps K, Pantazis C, Perrine SP. Erythroid progenitor proliferation is stimulated by phenoxyacetic and phenylalkyl acids. Blood Cells Mol Dis. 1996; 22 (2):150-8.

[115] Mankidy R, Faller DV, Mabaera R, Lowrey CH, Boosalis MS, White GL, Castaneda SA, Perrine SP. Short-chain fatty acids induce gamma-globin gene expression by displacement of a HDAC3-NCoR repressor complex. Blood. 2006; 108(9):3179-86.

[116] Noyer-Weidner M, Trautner TA. Methylation of DNA in prokaryotes. EXS. 1993; 64:39-108.

[117] Momparler RL, Eliopoulos N, Ayoub J. Evaluation of an inhibitor of DNA methylation, 5-aza-2'-deoxycytidine, for the treatment of lung cancer and the future role of gene therapy. Adv Exp Med Biol. 2000; 465:433-46.

[118] Robertson KD. DNA methylation, methyltransferases, and cancer. Oncogene. 2001; 20(24):3139-55.

[119] van der Ploeg LH, Flavell RA. DNA methylation in the human gamma delta beta-globin locus in erythroid and nonerythroid tissues. Cell. 1980; 19(4):947-58.

[120] Torrealba de Ron A, Papayannopoulou T, Stamatoyannopoulos G. Studies of Hb F in adult nonanemic baboons: Hb F expression in erythroid colonies decreases as the level of maturation of Erythroid progenitors advances. Exp Hematol. 1985; 13:919-925.

[121] DeSimone J, Koshy M, Dorn L, Lavelle D, Bressler L, Molokie R, Talischy N. Maintenance of elevated fetal hemoglobin levels by decitabine during dose interval treatment of sickle cell anemia. Blood. 2002; 99(11):3905-8.

[122] Saunthararajah Y, DeSimone J. Clinical studies with fetal hemoglobin-enhancing agents in sickle cell disease. Semin Hematol. 2004; 41(46):11-6.

[123] Lavelle DE. The molecular mechanism of fetal hemoglobin reactivation. Semin Hematol. 2004; 41:3-10.

[124] DeSimone J, Heller P, Hall L, Zwiers D. 5-Azacytidine stimulates fetal hemoglobin synthesis in anemic baboons. Proc Natl Acad Sci U S A. 1982; 79:4428-4431.

[125] Ley TJ, DeSimone J, Anagnou NP, Keller GH, Humphries RK, Turner PH, Young NS, Keller P, Nienhuis AW. 5-azacytidine selectively increases gamma-globin synthesis in a patient with $beta^{+}$ thalassemia. N Engl J Med. 1982; 307(24):1469-75.

[126] Carr BI, Reilly JG, Smith SS, Winberg C, Riggs A. The tumorigenicity of 5-azacytidine in the male Fischer rat. Carcinogenesis. 1984; 5:1583-1590.

[127] Hermes M, Osswald H, Kloor D. Role of S-adenosylhomocysteine hydrolase in adenosine-induced apoptosis in HepG2 cells. Exp Cell Res. 2007; 313(2):264-83.

[128] He M, Fan J, Jiang R, Tang WX, Wang ZW. Expression of DNMTs and genomic DNA methylation in gastric signet ring cell carcinoma. Mol Med Rep. 2013; 8(3):942-8.

[129] Rupon JW, Wang SZ, Gaensler K, Lloyd J, Ginder GD. Methyl binding domain protein 2 mediates gamma-globin gene silencing in adult human betaYAC transgenic mice. Proc Natl Acad Sci U S A. 2006; 103(17):6617-22.

[130] Chin MH, Mason MJ, Xie W, Volinia S, Singer M, Peterson C, Ambartsumyan G, Aimiuwu O, Richter L, Zhang J, Khvorostov I, Ott V, Grunstein M, Lavon N, Benvenisty N, Croce CM, Clark AT, Baxter T, Pyle AD, Teitell MA, Pelegrini M, Plath K, Lowry WE. Induced pluripotent stem cells and embryonic stem cells are distinguished by gene expression signatures. Cell Stem Cell. 2009; 5(1):111-23.

[131] Bauer S, Robinson PN, Gagneur J. Model-based gene set analysis for Bioconductor. Bioinformatics. 2011; 27: 1882-1883.

[132] Turner B.M. Histone acetylation and control of gene expression. J. Cell Science. 1991; 99:13-20.

[133] Hassig CA, Schreiber SL. Nuclear histone acetylases and deacetylases and transcriptional regulation: HATs off to HDACs. Curr Opin Chem Biol. 1997; 1(3):300-8.

[134] Mizzen CA, Allis CD. Linking histone acetylation to transcriptional regulation. Cell Mol Life Sci. 1998; 54(1):6-20.

[135] Kuo MH, Allis CD. Roles of histone acetyltransferases and deacetylases in gene regulation. Bioessays. 1998; 20(8):615-26.

[136] Felsenfeld G, Groudine M. Controlling the double helix. Nature. 2003; 421(6921): 448-53.

[137] Glozak MA, Sengupta N, Zhang X, Seto E. Acetylation and deacetylation of non-histone proteins. Gene. 2005; 363:15-23.

[138] Yang XJ, Seto E. HATs and HDACs: from structure, function and regulation to novel strategies for therapy and prevention. Oncogene. 2007; 26(37):5310-8.

[139] Smith CL. A shifting paradigm: histone deacetylases and transcriptional activation. Bioessays. 2008; 30(1):15-24.

[140] Dokmanovic M, Clarke C, Marks PA. Histone deacetylase inhibitors: overview and perspectives. Mol Cancer Res. 2007; 5(10):981-9.

[141] Seto E, Yoshida M. Erasers of histone acetylation: the histone deacetylase enzymes. Cold Spring Harb Perspect Biol. 2014; 6(4):018713.

[142] Imai S, Armstrong CM, Kaeberlein M, Guarente L-Transcriptional silencing and longevity protein Sir2 is an NAD-dependent histone deacetylase. Nature. 2000; 403:795-800.

[143] Verdin E, Dequiedt F, Kasler HG. Class II histone deacetylases: versatile regulators. Trends Genet. 2003; 19(5):286-93.

[144] Forsberg EC, Downs KM, Christensen HM, Im H, Nuzzi PA, Bresnick EH. Developmentally dynamic histone acetylation pattern of a tissue-specific chromatin domain. Proc Natl Acad Sci U S A. 2000; 97(26):14494-9.

[145] Mai A, Massa S, Rotili D, Cerbara I, Valente S, Pezzi R, Simeoni S, Ragno R. Histone deacetylation in epigenetics: an attractive target for anticancer therapy. Med Res Rev. 2005; 25(3):261-309.

[146] Martin DG, Grimes DE, Baetz K, Howe L. Methylation of histone H3 mediates the association of the NuA3 histone acetyltransferase with chromatin. Mol Cell Biol. 2006; 26:3018-3028.

[147] Shalini A. Muralidhar, Valya Ramakrishnan, Inderdeep S. Kalra, Wei Li, Betty S. Pace. Histone Deacetylase 9 Activates γ-Globin Gene Expression in Primary ErythroidCells. J Biol Chem. 2011; 286(3):2343-2353.

[148] Skarpidi E, Vassilopoulos G, Li Q, Stamatoyannopoulos G. Novel in vitro assay for the detection of pharmacologic inducers of fetal hemoglobin. Blood. 2000; 96:321-326.

[149] Makala L, Di Maro S, Lou TF, Sivanand S, Ahn JM, Pace BS. FK228 Analogues Induce Fetal Hemoglobin in Human Erythroid Progenitors. Anemia. 2012; 2012:428137.

[150] Bradner JE, Mak R, Tanguturi SK, Mazitschek R, Haggarty SJ, Ross K, Chang CY, Bosco J, West N, Morse E, Lin K, Shen JP, Kwiatkowski NP, Gheldof N, Dekker J, DeAngelo DJ, Carr SA, Schreiber SL, Golub TR, Ebert BL. Chemical genetic strategy identifies histone deacetylase 1 (HDAC1) and HDAC2 as therapeutic targets in sickle cell disease. Proc Natl Acad Sci U S A. 2010; 107(28):12617-22.

[151] Shearstone JR vDJ, Bradner JE, Mazitschek R, Jones SS, Jarpe M. Induction of Human Fetal Hemoglobin Expression by Selective Inhibitors of Hilstone Deacetylase 1 and 2 (HDAC 1/2). Blood. 2012; 120:3259.

[152] Kappos L, Gold R, Arnold DL, Bar-Or A, Giovannoni G, Selmaj K, Sarda SP, Agarwal S, Zhang A, Sheikh SI, Seidman E, Dawson KT. Quality of life outcomes with BG-12 (dimethyl fumarate) in patients with relapsing-remitting multiple sclerosis: the DEFINE study. Mult Scler. 2014; 20(2):243-52.

[153] Macari ER, Schaeffer EK, West RJ, Lowrey CH. Simvastatin and t-butylhydroquinone suppress KLF1 and BCL11A gene expression and additively increase fetal hemoglobin in primary human erythroid cells. Blood. 2013; 121:830-839.

[154] Fox RJ, Kita M, Cohan SL, Henson LJ, Zambrano J, Scannevin RH, O'Gorman J, Novas M, Dawson KT, Phillips JT. BG-12 (dimethyl fumarate): a review of mechanism of action, efficacy, and safety. Curr Med Res Opin. 2014; 30(2):251-62.

[155] Makala L, Promsote W, Li B, Ganapathy V, Pamela M, Pace BS. Monomethylfumarate (MMF), a Novel Inducer of Fetal Hemoglobin in Human Erythroid Progenitors and Retinal Pigment Epithelial Cells.. Blood. 2013; 122:317.

[156] Menzel S, Garner C, Gut I, Matsuda F, Yamaguchi M, Heath S, Foglio M, Zelenika D, Boland A, Rooks H, Best S, Spector TD, Farrall M, Lathrop M, Thein SL. A QTL influencing F cell production maps to a gene encoding a zinc-finger protein on chromosome 2p15. Nat Genet. 2007; 39(10):1197-9.

[157] Townes TM, Behringer RR. Human globin locus activation region (LAR): role in temporal control. Trends Genet. 1990; 6:219-223.

[158] Ryan TM, Ciavatta DJ, Townes TM. Knockout-transgenic mouse model of sickle cell disease. Science. 1997; 278:873-876.

[159] Meiler SE, Wade M, Kutlar F, Yerigenahally SD, Xue Y, Moutouh-de Parseval LA, Corral LG, Swerdlow PS, Kutlar A. Pomalidomide augments fetal hemoglobin production without the myelosuppressive effects of hydroxyurea in transgenic sickle cell mice. Blood. 2011; 118(4):1109-12.

[160] Shi Y, Lan F, Matson C, Mulligan P, Whetstine JR, Cole PA, Casero RA, Shi Y. Histone demethylation mediated by the nuclear amine oxidase homolog LSD1. Cell. 2004; 119(7):941-53.

[161] Shi L, Cui S, Engel JD, Tanabe O. Lysine-specific demethylase 1 is a therapeutic target for fetal hemoglobin induction. Nat Med. 2013; 19:291-294.

[162] Platt OS, Orkin SH, Dover G, Beardsley GP, Miller B, Nathan DG. Hydroxyurea enhances fetal hemoglobin production in sickle cell anemia. J Clin Invest. 1984; 74:652-656.

[163] Charache S, Terrin ML, Moore RD, Dover GJ, Barton FB, Eckert SV, McMahon RP, Bonds DR. Effect of hydroxyurea on the frequency of painful crises in sickle cell anemia. Investigators of the Multicenter Study of Hydroxyurea in Sickle Cell Anemia. N Engl J Med. 1995; 332(20):1317-22.

[164] Steinberg MH, Lu ZH, Barton FB, Terrin ML, Charache S, Dover GJ. Fetal hemoglobin in sickle cell anemia: determinants of response to hydroxyurea. Multicenter Study of Hydroxyurea. Blood. 1997; 89:1078-1088.

[165] Moore RD, Charache S, Terrin ML, Barton FB, Ballas SK. Cost effectiveness of hydroxyurea in sickle cell anemia. Investigators of the Multicenter Study of Hydroxyurea in Sickle Cell Anemia. Am J Hematol. 2000; 64:26-31.

[166] Steinberg MH, McCarthy WF, Castro O, Ballas SK, Armstrong FD, Smith W, Ataga K, Swerdlow P, Kutlar A, DeCastro L, Waclawiw MA. Investigators of the Multicenter Study of Hydroxyurea in Sickle Cell Anemia and MSH Patients' Follow-Up. The risks and benefits of long-term use of hydroxyurea in sickle cell anemia: A 17.5 year follow-up. Am J Hematol. 2010; 85(6):403-8.

[167] Voskaridou E, Christoulas D, Bilalis A, Plata E, Varvagiannis K, Stamatopoulos G, Sinopoulou K, Balassopoulou A, Loukopoulos D, Terpos E. The effect of prolonged administration of hydroxyurea on morbidity and mortality in adult patients with sickle cell syndromes: results of a 17-year, single-center trial (LaSHS). Blood. 2010; 115(12): 2354-63.

[168] Wang WC, Wynn LW, Rogers ZR, Scott JP, Lane PA, Ware RE. A two year pilot trial of hydroxyurea in very young children with sickle cell anemia. J Pediatr. 2001; 139:790-796.

[169] Hankins JS, Ware RE, Rogers ZR, Wynn LW, Lane PA, Scott JP, Wang WC. Long-term hydroxyurea therapy for infants with sickle cell anemia: the HUSOFT extension study. Blood. 2005; 106(7):2269-75.

[170] Wang WC1, Ware RE, Miller ST, Iyer RV, Casella JF, Minniti CP, Rana S, Thornburg CD, Rogers ZR, Kalpatthi RV, Barredo JC, Brown RC, Sarnaik SA, Howard TH, Wynn LW, Kutlar A, Armstrong FD, Files BA, Goldsmith JC, Waclawiw MA, Huang X, Thompson BW; BABY HUG investigators. Hydroxycarbamide in very young children with sickle cell anaemia: a multicentre, randomised, controlled trial (BABY HUG). Lancet. 2011; 377(9778):1663-72.

[171] Zimmerman SA, Schultz WH, Burgett S, Mortier NA, Ware RE. Hydroxyurea therapy lowers transcranial Doppler flow velocities in children with sickle cell anemia. Blood. 2007; 110:1043-1047.

[172] Hankins JS, Helton KJ, McCarville MB, Li CS, Wang WC, Ware RE. Preservation of spleen and brain function in children with sickle cell anemia treated with hydroxyurea. Pediatr Blood Cancer. 2008; 50:293-297.

[173] Thornburg CD, Dixon N, Burgett S, Mortier NA, Schultz WH, Zimmerman SA, Bonner M, Hardy KK, Calatroni A, Ware RE. A pilot study of hydroxyurea to prevent chronic organ damage in young children with sickle cell anemia. Pediatr Blood Cancer. 2009; 52(5):609-15.

[174] Ware RE, Schultz WH, Yovetich N, Mortier NA, Alvarez O, Hilliard L, Iyer RV, Miller ST, Rogers ZR, Scott JP, Waclawiw M, Helms RW. Stroke With Transfusions Changing to Hydroxyurea (SWiTCH): a phase III randomized clinical trial for treatment of children with sickle cell anemia, stroke, and iron overload. Pediatr Blood Cancer. 2011; 57(6):1011-7.

[175] Ware RE, Helms RW, SWiTCH Investigators. Stroke With Transfusions Changing to Hydroxyurea (SWiTCH). Blood. 2012; 119:3925-3932.

[176] Noel N, Ko C. Natural Remedies for the Treatment of Beta-Thalassemia and Sickle Cell Anemia—Current Status and Perspectives in Fetal Hemoglobin Reactivation. Hindawi Publishing Corporation International Scholarly Research Notices. Volume 2014, (123257): 11.

[177] Heinrich M, Gibbons S. Ethnopharmacology in drug discovery: an analysis of its role and potential contribution. J Pharm Pharmacol. 2001; 53:425-32.

[178] Khan MT, Lampronti I, Martello D, Bianchi N, Jabbar S, Choudhuri MS, et al. Identification of pyrogallol as an antiproliferative compound present in extracts from the

medicinal plant Emblica officinalis: effects on in vitro cell growth of human tumor cell lines.Int J Oncol. 2002; 21:187-92.

[179] Lampronti I, Martello D, Bianchi N, Borgatti M, Lambertini E, Piva R, Jabbar S, Choudhuri MS, Khan MT, Gambari R. In vitro antiproliferative effects on human tumor cell lines of extracts from the Bangladeshi medicinal plant Aegle marmelos Correa. Phytomedicine. 2003; 10(4):300-8.

[180] Lambertini E, Piva R, Khan MT, Lampronti I, Bianchi N, Borgatti M, Gambari R. Effects of extracts from Bangladeshi medicinal plants on in vitro proliferation of human breast cancer cell lines and expression of estrogen receptor alpha gene. Int J Oncol. 2004; 24(2):419-23.

[181] Xie F, Wu CF, Lai WP, Yang XJ, Cheung PY, Yao XS, Leung PC, Wong MS. The osteoprotective effect of Herba epimedii (HEP) extract in vivo and in vitro. Evid Based Complement Alternat Med. 2005; 2(3):353-61.

[182] Saad B, Azaizeh H, Said O. Tradition and perspectives of arab herbal medicine: a review. Evid Based Complement Alternat Med. 2005;2:475-9.

[183] Lampronti I, Khan MT, Bianchi N, Ather A, Borgatti M, Vizziello L, Fabbri E, Gambari R. Bangladeshi medicinal plant extracts inhibiting molecular interactions between nuclear factors and target DNA sequences mimicking NF-kappaB binding sites. Med Chem. 2005; 1(4):327-33.

[184] Adams LS, Seeram NP, Hardy ML, Carpenter C, Heber D. Analysis of the interactions of botanical extract combinations against the viability of prostate cancer cell lines. Evid Based Complement Alternat Med. 2006; 3:117-24.

[185] Luo JZ, Luo L. American ginseng stimulates insulin production and prevents apoptosis through regulation of uncoupling Protein-2 in cultured beta cells. Evid Based Complement Alternat Med 2006; 3:365-72.

[186] Jagetia GC, Rao SK. Evaluation of cytotoxic effects of dichloromethane extract of guduchi (Tinospora cordifoliaMiers ex Hook F & THOMS) on cultured HeLa cells. Evid Based Complement Alternat Med. 2006; 3:267-72.

[187] Guerrini A, Lampronti I, Bianchi N, Zuccato C, Breveglieri G, Salvatori F, Mancini I, Rossi D, Potenza R, Chiavilli F, Sacchetti G, Gambari R, Borgatti M. Bergamot (Citrus bergamia Risso) fruit extracts as γ-globin gene expression inducers: phytochemical and functional perspectives. J Agric Food Chem. 2009; 57(10):4103-11.

[188] H. Li , C. H. Ko, S. Y. Tsang, P. C. Leung, M. C. Fung, and K. P. Fung., The ethanol extract of Fructus trichosanthis promotes fetal hemoglobin production via p38 MAPK activation and Erk inactivation in K562 cells. Evidence-Based Complementary and Alternative Medicine, vol. 2011, Article ID 657056, 8.

[189] Fibach E, Bianchi N, Borgatti M, Prus E, Gambari R. Mithramycin induces fetal hemoglobin production in normal and thalassemic human erythroid precursor cells. Blood. 2003; 102(4):1276-81.

[190] Menzel S1, Garner C, Gut I, Matsuda F, Yamaguchi M, Heath S, Foglio M, Zelenika D, Boland A, Rooks H, Best S, Spector TD, Farrall M, Lathrop M, Thein SL. A QTL influencing F cell production maps to a gene encoding a zinc-finger protein on chromosome 2p15. Nat Genet. 2007; 39(10):1197-9.

[191] Thein SL, Menzel S. Discovering the genetics underlying foetal haemoglobin production in adults. Br J Haematol. 2009; 145:455-467.

[192] van der Ploeg LH, Flavell RA. DNA methylation in the human gamma delta beta-globin locus in erythroid and nonerythroid tissues. Cell. 1980; 19:947-958.

[193] Letvin NL, Linch DC, Beardsley GP, McIntyre KW, Nathan DG. Augmentation of fetal-hemoglobin production in anemic monkeys by hydroxyurea. N Engl J Med. 1984; 310:869-873.

[194] DeSimone J, Heller P, Molokie RE, Hall L, Zwiers D. Tetrahydrouridine, cytidine analogues, and hemoglobin F. Am J Hematol. 1985; 18:283-288.

[195] Saunthararajah Y, Hillery CA, Lavelle D, Molokie R, Dorn L, Bressler L, Gavazova S, Chen YH, Hoffman R, DeSimone J. Effects of 5-aza-2'-deoxycytidine on fetal hemoglobin levels, red cell adhesion, and hematopoietic differentiation in patients with sickle cell disease. Blood. 2003; 102(12):3865-70.

[196] Lavelle D, Chin J, Vaitkus K, Redkar S, Phiasivongsa P, Tang C, Will R, Hankewych M, Roxas B, Singh M, Saunthararajah Y, Desimone J. Oral decitabine reactivates expression of the methylated gamma-globin gene in Papio anubis. Am J Hematol. 2007; 82(11):981-5.

[197] Inati A, Kahale M, Perrine SP, Chui DH, Taher AT, Koussa S, Abi Nasr T, Abbas HA, Ghalie RG. A phase 2 study of HQK-1001, an oral fetal haemoglobin inducer, in β-thalassaemia intermedia. Br J Haematol. 2014; 164(3):456-8.

[198] Peterson KR, Navas PA, Stamatoyannopoulos G. beta-YAC transgenic mice for studying LCR function. Ann N Y Acad Sci. 1998; 850:28-37.

[199] Johnson J, Hunter R, McElveen R, Qian XH, Baliga BS, Pace BS. Fetal hemoglobin induction by the histone deacetylase inhibitor, scriptaid. Cell Mol Biol (Noisy-le-grand). 2005; 51:229-238.

[200] Moore RD, Charache S, Terrin ML, Barton FB, Ballas SK. Costeffectiveness of hydroxyurea in sickle cell anemia. Investigators of the Multicenter Study of Hydroxyurea in Sickle Cell Anemia. Am J Hematol. 2000; 64:26-31.

[201] Lanzkron S, Haywood C Jr, Segal JB, Dover GJ. Hospitalization rates and costs of care of patients with sickle cell anemia in the state of Maryland in the era of hydroxyurea. Am J Hematol. 2006; 81:927-932.

[202] Walters MC1, Storb R, Patience M, Leisenring W, Taylor T, Sanders JE, Buchanan GE, Rogers ZR, Dinndorf P, Davies SC, Roberts IA, Dickerhoff R, Yeager AM, Hsu L, Kurtzberg J, Ohene-Frempong K, Bunin N, Bernaudin F, Wong WY, Scott JP, Margolis D, Vichinsky E, Wall DA, Wayne AS, Pegelow C, Redding-Lallinger R, Wiley J, Klemperer M, Mentzer WC, Smith FO, Sullivan KM. Impact of bone marrow transplantation for symptomatic sickle cell disease: An interim report. Multicenter investigation of bone marrow transplantation for sickle cell disease. Blood. 2000 Mar; 95(6): 1918-24.

[203] Locatelli F, Rocha V, Reed W, Bernaudin F, Ertem M, Grafakos S, Brichard B, Li X, Nagler A, Giorgiani G, Haut PR, Brochstein JA, Nugent DJ, Blatt J, Woodard P, Kurtzberg J, Rubin CM, Miniero R, Lutz P, Raja T, Roberts I, Will AM, Yaniv I, Vermylen C, Tannoia N, Garnier F, Ionescu I, Walters MC, Lubin BH, Gluckman E; Eurocord Transplant Group. Related umbilical cord blood transplantation in patients with thalassemia and sickle cell disease. Blood. 2003; 101(6):2137-43.

[204] Kharbanda S, Smith AR, Hutchinson SK, McKenna DH, Ball JB, Lamb LS Jr, Agarwal R, Weinberg KI, Wagner JE Jr. Unrelated donor allogeneic hematopoietic stem cell transplantation for patients with hemoglobinopathies using a reduced-intensity conditioning regimen and third-party mesenchymal stromal cells. Biol Blood Marrow Transplant. 2014; 20(4):581-6.

[205] Cavazzana-Calvo M, Payen E, Negre O, Wang G, Hehir K, Fusil F, Down J, Denaro M, Brady T, Westerman K, Cavallesco R, Gillet-Legrand B, Caccavelli L, Sgarra R, Maouche-Chrétien L, Bernaudin F, Girot R, Dorazio R, Mulder GJ, Polack A, Bank A, Soulier J, Larghero J, Kabbara N, Dalle B, Gourmel B, Socie G, Chrétien S, Cartier N, Aubourg P, Fischer A, Cornetta K, Galacteros F, Beuzard Y, Gluckman E, Bushman F, Hacein-Bey-Abina S, Leboulch P. Transfusion independence and HMGA2 activation after gene therapy of human β-thalassaemia. Nature. 2010; 467(7313):318-22.

[206] Leboulch P. Gene therapy: primed for take-off. Nature. 2013; 500:280-282.

[207] Takahashi K, Yamanaka S. Induction of pluripotent stem cells from mouse embryonic and adult fibroblast cultures by defined factors. Cell. 2006; 126:663-676.

[208] Hanna J, Wernig M, Markoulaki S, Sun CW, Meissner A, Cassady JP, Beard C, Brambrink T, Wu LC, Townes TM, Jaenisch R. Treatment of sickle cell anemia mouse model with iPS cells generated from autologous skin. Science. 2007; 318(5858):1920-3.

[209] Yu J, Vodyanik MA, Smuga-Otto K, Antosiewicz-Bourget J, Frane JL, Tian S, Nie J, Jonsdottir GA, Ruotti V, Stewart R, Slukvin II, Thomson JA. Induced pluripotent stem cell lines derived from human somatic cells. Science. 2007; 318(5858):1917-20.

Chapter 8

Novel Therapy Approaches in β-Thalassemia Syndromes — A Role of Genetic Modifiers

Sonja Pavlovic, Milena Ugrin and Maja Stojiljkovic

Additional information is available at the end of the chapter

http://dx.doi.org/10.5772/61023

Abstract

The β-thalassemia syndromes are heterogeneous autosomal recessive hereditary disorders, caused by alterations in the *HBB* gene and characterized by absent or reduced β-globin chain synthesis. The β-thalassemia phenotypes are variable, ranging from severe, transfusion-dependent thalassemia major to mild, asymptomatic thalassemia trait. This interpatient clinical variability has swayed researchers toward identifying genetic modifiers for these disorders. Primary modifiers refer to type of alterations affecting β-globin gene. Secondary modifiers include variations in genes affecting α/β-globin chain equilibrium, such as genes involved in the γ-globin gene expression and genes affecting the amount and stability of α-globin chains. Tertiary modifiers are gene variations affecting the phenotype with regard to the complications caused by β-thalassemia syndromes. A role of secondary genetic modifiers in ameliorating the clinical phenotype has been observed. Secondary genetic modifiers are the most common targets for modern therapy and could be located within α- and γ-globin genes or outside globin gene cluster. The most potent secondary modifier genes are γ-globin genes. Production of fetal hemoglobin (HbF) trough adulthood ameliorates the severity of β-thalassemia phenotype. Large family and genome-wide association studies have shown that regions outside of the β-globin gene cluster are also implicated in γ-globin gene expression regulation. *HBS1-MYB* intragenic region and *BCL11A* gene have been particularly studied. Variants within these loci, along with γ-globin gene variants, account for approximately 50% of the HbF level variation, suggesting that additional factors are involved (transcription regulators (KLF1), regulators of α-globin chain stability (AHSP), epigenetic regulators (FoP)). Until recently a definitive cure for β-thalassemia could be achieved with bone marrow transplantation. However, it is available for less than 30% of the patients and bears a significant risk of morbidity and mortality. Alternative strategies, such as gene therapy and development of induced pluripotent stem cells (iPSCs) have been explored. The targets for gene therapy are hematopoietic stem cells, which are harvested from patient bone marrow or peripheral blood, purified by immunoselection, transduced by "therapeutic gene" aimed at correcting the effect of defective β-globin gene, and returned to the patient. Various types of vectors have been considered for gene transfer, including non viral (tRNK and ribozymes) and viral (retroviral and lentiviral vectors). In the past few years, iPSCs emerged as an interesting candidate for gene transfer. The feature that makes these cells appealing in the field of gene therapy is their susceptibility to gene correction by homologous recombination. Therapy protocols based on molecular basis of β-thalassemia are the best example of novel approaches in disease treatment.

Keywords: β-thalassemia, modifier genes, gene therapy, iPSC

---

1. Introduction

1.1. Hemoglobinopathies

Hemoglobinopathies are very heterogenic group of hereditary anemias and are classified according to the qualitative nature of the resulting hemoglobin and the quantitative amount of hemoglobin produced.

"Qualitative" hemoglobinopathies, or structural hemoglobin variants, are characterized by amino acid sequence variation of the hemoglobin (Hb) molecule which influences biochemical features of Hb. "Quantitative" hemoglobin disorders or thalassemias, are classified according to the deficient globin chain and, hence, include α-thalassemia and β-thalassemia.

Moreover, there is a distinct group of disorders classified as β -thalassemia syndromes which comprises β-thalassemia and certain group of hemoglobin variants whose synthesis is reduced due to amino acid sequence variation in the regions responsible for regulation of transcription or peptide stability.

Molecular mechanisms leading to formation of "quantitative" Hb variants include a δ-β hybrid gene (Hb Lepore) [1] and mutations causing hyperunstable beta globin chain synthesis (Hb Sabine) [2]. These highly unstable Hb variants precipitate before assembling with the α-globin chains to produce the Hb tetramer, resulting in excess of the α-globin chains and, thus, ineffective erythropoiesis [3, 4].

1.2. β-thalassemia syndromes

The β-thalassemia syndromes are one of the most common autosomal recessive hereditary disorders worldwide, with high prevalence in the populations of the Mediterranean, Middle-East, Central Asia, Indian subcontinent and Far East [3]. The β-thalassemias are caused by alterations in the β-globin gene and characterized by absent (β^0-thalassemia) or reduced (β^+-

thalassemia) synthesis of β-globin chain of adult hemoglobin (HbA; $\alpha_2\beta_2$). The result of this reduced globin chain synthesis is reduced production of functional hemoglobin tetramers which leads to hypochromia (decrease in the hemoglobin content of the erythrocytes) and microcytosis (reduces mean corpuscular volume of erythrocytes). Also, the excess of unbound α-globin chains precipitate in erythroid precursors in the bone marrow and red blood cells in circulation, leading to their premature death and, hence, to ineffective erythropoiesis and hemolytic anemia [5].

The clinical manifestations of β-thalassemias are extremely diverse, ranging form the severe, transfusion-dependent thalassemia major to the mild, asymptomatic thalassemia trait. Diverse phenotypes between the two extremes of thalassemia major and thalassemia trait constitute the clinical syndrome of thalassemia intermedia [6].

1.3. β-globin gene locus

The β-globin gene (*HBB*) maps in the short arm of chromosome 11, in the 70 kb region that also contains four other functional globin genes: embryonic, ε-globin gene (*HBE*), the fetal $^{A}\gamma$- and $^{G}\gamma$-globin genes (*HBG1* and *HBG2*) and adult δ-globin gene (*HBD*) as well as ψβ pseudogene. The five functional globin genes are arranged in the order of their developmental expression [7]. Upstream of the β globin complex is the locus control region (LCR), important regulatory region which consists of five erythroid-specific DNase1 hypersensitive (HS) sites (HS 1–5) distributed between 6 and 20 kb 5′ of the ε-globin gene (Fig.1). These HS sites interact with each other and two additional 5′ and one 3′ HSs to form an active chromatin hub (ACH) through looping, which interacts with the specific globin gene in any given moment of development. The role of the individual HS is still unclear, although HS2 and HS3 appear to be the most important sites for the efficiency of transcription, each leading to an ~30% loss of transcription when deleted [6, 8].

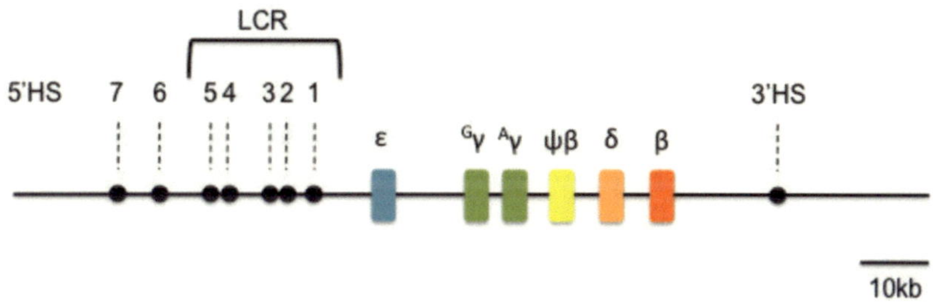

Figure 1. Structure of β-globin gene cluster. Human β-globin gene locus showing embryonic (ε), fetal ($^{A}\gamma$;$^{G}\gamma$) and adult (δ;β) globin genes, controlled by locus control region (LCR) and additional hypersensitive sites (3'HS; 5'HS). Region between fetal and adult globin gene contains ψβ pseudogene. The five functional globin genes are arranged in the order of their developmental expression.

During fetal development and the first six months of neonatal life, a complex pattern of globin gene expression occurs called the hemoglobin switch. Namely, in the early part of the first trimester, there is high expression of an embryonic globin gene within the primitive lineage of erythrocytes in the yolk sac. During fetal development, however, predominantly expressed globin genes are γ-globin genes, coding for the γ-globin polypeptides, produced within fetal liver. These γ-globin chains combine with adult α-globin chains into a stable tetramer forming fetal hemoglobin (HbF; $\alpha_2\gamma_2$). Shortly after the time of birth this fetal hemoglobin is progressively replaced by the adult hemoglobin (HbA), which is mediated by a transcriptional switch in definitive erythroid progenitors from γ- to β-globin [9, 10].

2. Genetic modifiers of β-thalassemia

The β-thalassemia is caused by more than 200 point mutations and, rarely, by deletions [11]. However, genotypic variability at known loci is often insufficient to explain the phenotypic variability between individuals with the same genotype [12]. This interpatient clinical variability in the β-thalassemia syndromes has swayed researchers toward identifying genetic modifiers of severity for these disorders. Such genetic modifiers could potentially lead to the development of more specific and effective therapies [13]. Genetic modifiers exert their potential on three levels: primary, secondary and tertiary.

Primary modifiers usually refer to a type of alterations affecting β-globin gene. Location of the mutations within different gene regions determines the phenotypic severity, therefore the point mutations affecting the β-globin expression belong to three different categories: mutations leading to defective β-globin gene transcription (promoter and 5′ UTR mutations); mutations affecting mRNA processing (splice-junction and consensus sequence mutations, polyadenylation, and other 3′ UTR mutations); and mutations resulting in abnormal mRNA translation (nonsense, frameshift, and initiation codon mutations) [3]. Mutations affecting transcription usually result in a mild deficit of β-globin production that reflects the relatively mild phenotype of these β^+-thalassemias. The example of transcription affecting mutation is the C>T mutation at position -101 to the β-globin gene which appears to cause an extremely mild deficit of β-globin, such that it is asymptomatic in heterozygotes who have normal HbA_2 ($\alpha_2\delta_2$) levels [6]. Mutations affecting β-globin mRNA processing are located within 5′- and 3′-splice junction (donor and acceptor site), as well as within splice junctions′ consensus sequences. Mutations altering the donor and acceptor splice site lead to deficiency of functional mRNA production resulting in complete absence of β-globin polypeptide chains and, hence, to β^0-thalassemia. On the other hand, mutations affecting consensus sequences surrounding splice-junction, decrease the efficiency of the normal splicing to varying degrees, hence producing β-thalassemia phenotype that ranges from mild to severe [7]. Also, these mutations could affect cryptic splice site, sequence that mimics a consensus sequence, leading to low efficiency splicing and therefore milder form of β-thalassemia. Cap-site mutations, as well as mutations affecting polyadenylation also lead to mild, β^+-thalassemia phenotype [14]. Mutations disrupting the mRNA translation ether in initiation or elongation phase, result in β^0-thalassemia phenotype. Most of these defects result from the introduction of premature termination codons due to frameshift or nonsense mutations and nearly all terminate within first and second exon [15].

Secondary modifiers include variations in genes affecting α/β globin chain equilibrium such as α- and γ-globin genes, as well as genes involved in the γ-globin gene expression (*HBS1-*

MYB, BCL11A, KLF1, C1orf77) and genes affecting the amount and stability of α-globin chains (*AHSP*). These genetic modifiers could be located within (α- and γ-globin genes) or outside globin gene cluster. In the recent years, there has been significant advancement in the fields of secondary genetic modifiers ameliorating the clinical phenotype of β-thalassemia syndromes. Specifically, production of fetal hemoglobin (HbF) trough adulthood could ameliorate the severity of β-thalassemia phenotype since γ-globin polypeptide chains compensate for the lack of the functional β-globin polypeptide chains. This is why γ-globin genes, along with other secondary modifiers, represent the most common targets for modern therapeutic.

Tertiary modifiers are gene variations affecting the phenotype with regard to some of the complications caused by β-thalassemia syndromes such as hyperbilirubinemia, propensity to gallstone formation, bone diseases, thrombophilia and cardiopathies [6].

Hyperbilirubinemia and gallstone formation (cholelithiasis) is a common complication of β-thalassemia and is attributed to the rapid turnover of the red blood cells, bilirubin being a breakdown product of hemoglobin. It occurs with variable incidence in homozygous β-thalassemia with the reported variation being partly related to the age of the patients and to its clinical severity, as it is more common in thalassemia intermedia than thalassemia major. Studies have shown that the levels of bilirubin and the predisposition to gallstones in β-thalassemia is related to a polymorphic variant in the promoter of the uridine diphosphate-glucoronyltransferase A1 (*UGT1A1*) gene, also referred to as Gilbert's syndrome. Individuals who are homozygous for the this (TA)7 variant instead of the usual (TA)6, tend to have higher levels of bilirubin and increased predisposition to gallstone [16, 17].

Progressive osteoporosis and osteopenia is another increasingly common complication observed in young adults with β-thalassemia and it is determined by a combination of genetic and environmental factors. Anemia and bone marrow expansion which are prevalent in β-thalassemia are major contributors in inadequately treated patients. Bone mass, the main indicator of the osteoporosis and osteopenia, is another quantitative trait known to be under strong genetic control involving multiple loci including estrogen receptor gene, vitamin D receptor (*VDR*), collagen type a1 and type a2 genes (*COL1A1, COL1A2*), and transforming growth factor β1 (*TGFβ1*) [15].

The presence of a higher than normal incidence of thromboembolic events, mainly in β-thalassemia intermedia patients, and the existence of prothrombotic hemostatic anomalies in the majority of the patients, have led to the recognition of the existence of a chronic hyper-coagulable state in thalassemic patients [18]. Genetic risk factors for thrombosis, such as mutations in the gene for Factor II and Factor V, as well as variations in the *MTHFR* gene, could significantly influence the phenotype of the β-thalassemia syndromes [19].

Cardiac diseases are the main cause of death in β-thalassemia patients and are attributed to iron overload because of regular transfusions, increased iron intestinal absorption, and ineffective erythropoiesis during the life span of the patients. One of the studies depicted apolipoprotein E4 and it decreased antioxidant activity, as a risk factor for left ventricular failure (LVF) in thalassemia patients. However, the presence of this E4 allele does not guarantee the development of LVF in β-thalassemia but, when present, does affect the severity of the disease [20, 21].

3. Secondary genetic modifiers of β-thalassemia

3.1. Genetic modifiers of β-thalassemia within globin gene loci

3.1.1. α-globin genes

The α-globin genes encoding the α-globin chains are duplicated (α_1- and α_2-globin genes) and localized in the telomeric region of chromosome 16 (16p13.3), in a cluster containing also an embryonic, ζ-gene, encoding the embryonic globin chains, three pseudogenes (pseudo ζ-, pseudo α_1- and pseudo α_2-gene) and θ-gene of unknown function [22]. The level of transcription of the two α-globin genes differs, as the α_2 gene encodes two to three times more α-globin than α_1 gene. The different expression of the two α-globin genes has implications for the amount of hemoglobin variant present in carriers of α_1- or α_2-globin mutations and for the pathophysiology of the deletional and nondeletional forms of α-thalassemia [23]. As with β-thalassemia, α-thalassemias are characterized by absent (α^0-thalassemia) or reduced (α^+-thalassemia) production of α-globin chains, thus resulting in globin chain imbalance. The majority of the α-thalassemia defects result from deletions involving one or both α-globin genes on the same chromosome whereas point mutations affecting the functional expression of one of the two α-globin genes are not as common [24].

In many populations in which β-thalassemia is prevalent, α-thalassemia occurs at high frequency as well, resulting in coinheritance of both conditions. In these cases, homozygotes or compound heterozygotes for β-thalassemia will exert less severe phenotype since they would have less redundant α-globin chains. Therefore, the degree of amelioration of β-thalassemia phenotype depends on the severity of the β-thalassemia alleles and the number of functional α-globin genes. At one extreme, homozygous β-thalassemia patients who have only one functional α-globin gene, have thalassemia intermedia. On the other hand, the presence of increased α-globin product, as a result of triplicated or quadruplicated α-globin genes in β-thalassemia heterozygotes, increase the globin chain imbalance, converting a typically clinically asymptomatic state to that of thalassemia intermedia [25]. However, the phenotype of a single extra α gene (ααα/αα) with heterozygous β-thalassemia is more variable and depends on the severity of the β-thalassemia allele [26, 27].

3.1.2. γ -globin genes

As already discussed, after a brief period of embryonic globin gene expression, the γ-globin chain of fetal hemoglobin (HbF) is predominantly expressed for much of gestation. Shortly after the time of birth, γ-globin is progressively replaced by the β-globin chain of adult hemoglobin (HbA).This complex process of globin gene expression called hemoglobin switch, is clinically important because the persistence or reactivation of γ-globin gene expression could mitigate the severity of the symptoms caused by β-thalassemia syndromes [9, 10].

Hereditary persistence of fetal hemoglobin (HPFH) is a condition characterized by continued γ-globin gene expression and, therefore, synthesis of high levels of HbF (1.6-30%) during adult life without other hematological abnormalities in affected heterozygotes. Two major types of HPFH have been described. Very high levels of fetal hemoglobin synthesis and uniform distribution of HbF among all RBCs characterize pancellular HPFH. On the other hand, heterocellular HPFH results from inherited increase in the number of erythrocytes with persisting production of fetal hemoglobin, termed F cells [28, 29].

Pancellular HPFH could further be divided into two classes. The deletional HPFH is caused by large deletions 3′ to the γ-globin genes, removing δ- and β-globin genes and part of the γδ intergenic DNA. These deletions appear to bring enhancer sequences into the proximity of the remaining γ-globin genes or remove specific regulatory sequences that play role as silencing elements for γ-globin genes, which in both cases promote high expression of fetal globin genes [4, 30]. Nondeletional form of HPFH are usually the result of point mutations (including small deletions) 5′ from the *cap* site of γ-globin gene promoters [28]. These point mutations occur in transcription factor binding motifs in the γ-globin gene promoters, clustered in three regions, around positions -114 to -117, at -175, and from -195 to -202 nucleotide [31]. The first region contains distal CCAAT box, responsible for binding basal CP1 and CDP transcriptional factor and erythroid-specific GATA1 and NF-E3 transcriptional factors [32]. Region which contains mutation g.-175 T>C contains binding site for GATA1 transcriptional factor while mutations affecting -195 to -202 region alter the affinity for binding of the Sp1 transcriptional factor [33-35]. Recent studies on γ-globin gene promoter, showed the presence of mutations associated with HPFH, outside of the known, -202 to -110, region. Namely, mutation g.-567 C>G upstream of the γ^G-globin gene (*HBG2*) alters a GATA1 binding motif which acts as a silencer of *HBG2* and is, thus, associated with increased γ-globin gene expression in affected adults [36].

Heterocellular HPFH is usually a result of mutations outside the β-globin gene cluster, such as locus located in the X chromosome. Namely, it was shown that a locus controlling F-cell production (FCP locus) is localized on Xp22.2 [37]. Despite these original findings, Xp22.2 loci affecting HbF levels were not supported by later genome-wide association studies (GWAS) [38, 39]. In some cases, elevated levels of HbF are observed in otherwise normal individuals, while in others, high HbF levels become apparent only when erythroid stress-producing factors are present [4, 30].

One of the common genetic variants that has little effect in normal individuals but favors a higher HbF response in the conditions of erythroid stress is XmnI-γ^G (g.-158 C>T) variant. This may explain why the same mutations on different chromosomal backgrounds are associated with different clinical severity. However, the HbF response associated with the XmnI-γ^G site is usually moderate and may not be sufficient to explain the wide difference in phenotype observed in some cases [26, 40]. Also, numerous studies do not support this positive effect of XmnI-γ^G, as a sole determinant on γ-globin gene expression [41, 42], which makes this issue very controversial.

Recently, large family and genome-wide association studies have shown that regions outside of the β-globin gene cluster are also implicated in γ-globin gene expression and HbF regulation. Two of them have been particularly studied: *HBS1-MYB* intragenic region and *BCL11A* gene.

3.2. Genetic modifiers of β-thalassemia outside globin gene loci

3.2.1. HBS1L-MYB intragenic region

Variants within *HBS1L-MYB* intragenic region, located on chromosome 6q23, account for more than 20% of the HbF level variance in northern Europeans. Most of these variants are distributed within 79 kb long region, which consist of three linkage disequilibrium blocks, referred to as *HBS1L-MYB* intergenic polymorphism (HMIP) blocks 1, 2, and 3. A small number of the variants shown to display an especially strong association with the increased levels of HbF, are concentrated in 24 kb of HMIP block 2, located 33 kb upstream of *HBS1L* and 65 kb upstream of *MYB* and include polymorphisms rs28384513, rs9399137 and rs4895441 [43, 44]. Despite strong genetic evidence and extensive studies, a clear mechanism trough which these variants are causing variation in HbF levels has remained elusive, although the two flanking genes, *HBS1L* and *MYB* are candidate target genes. Namely, recent data suggest that this intragenic area contains GATA1 binding motifs and is thought to have properties of regulatory element [44].

HBS1L gene is thought to be housekeeping gene because it is ubiquitously expressed. The function of *HBS1L*, a possible member of the "GTPases" superfamily, in the red blood cell development, and therefore in the regulation of HbF levels, is not immediately apparent and could be manifested indirectly, through its effect on the expression of various cytokines and transcription factors that impact erythroid cell growth [38, 45]. On the other hand, *MYB* gene, encoding the c-MYB transcriptional factor, is a well known regulator of hematopoiesis and erythropoiesis. This transcriptional factor plays an essential role in controlling the erythroid cellular proliferation/differentiation and acts as a potent negative regulator of HbF expression, trough which other genes, such as miR-15a and miR-16-1, play a role in HbF level variations [46, 47].

Although 6q22–23 locus, containing *HBS1L-MYB* intragenic region, have been extensively studied for over a decade, not enough attention had been paid in regard to other positional candidate genes in this quantitative trait loci (QTL). These include phosphodiesterase 7 (*PDE7B*), mitogen-activated protein kinase kinase kinase 5 (*MAP3K5*), and peroxisomal biogeneses factor 7 (*PEX7*) genes with their SNPs showing strong association with different HbF levels [48]. It was shown that a short tandem repeat in the *MAP3K5* promoter, as well as intronic variations within both *MAP3K5* and *PDE7B* genes could be associated with lower HbF levels and thus, more severe β-thalassemia phenotype [49]. MAP3K5, encoded by *MAP3K5* gene, is a member of the MAPK family and, as such, a part of the MAPK pathway. This signaling cascade is one of the most important mechanisms for the cytoplasmic transduction of extracellular signals. As such, MAP3K5, has not been clearly associated with mechanisms governing erythropoiesis. On the other hand, *PDE7B* could be considered a strong modifier gene candidate given its high affinity and specificity for cAMP, which has an inhibitory effect on γ-globin expression and, thus, plays a role in fetal-to-adult globin gene switching [50].

3.2.2. *BCL11A gene*

BCL11A (B-cell CLL/lymphoma 11A) is transcriptional repressor expressed in most hematopoietic cells and critically important in the T and B cell development. BCL11A is a zinc-finger protein with usually a C2N2 zinc finger at the N-terminal, and six other Krüppel-like C2H2 zinc fingers near the C-terminal and it has at least 4 predicted isoforms (XS, S, L, XL) due to the alternative splicing. It is encoded by *BCL11A* gene, which spans over 102 kb on chromosome 2p16 [51]. Genome-wide association studies (GWAS) have demonstrated that a meaningful fraction of the variations in HbF levels is accounted for by variants within *BCL11A* gene [39]. More precisely, close to 15% of the phenotypic variation in the HbF levels could be explained by variations in intron 2 of the *BCL11A* gene, such as rs4671393 and rs11886868 [42, 43]. Further, it was shown that BCL11A (L and XL isoforms) acts as a potent silencer of γ-globin gene expression [52] by binding not to γ-globin gene promoter, but to LCR and γ^{A}-δ intragenic region with known role in repression of fetal globin genes [53]. Its role as a repressor, BCL11A most probably exerts trough association with various partners within erythroid multiprotein complexes, including the repressive nucleosome remodeling and deacetylase complex (NuRD), GATA1, the erythroid master regulator, and SOX6, a transcription factor previously shown to repress embryonic globin genes in mice [54]. Evidence that BCL11A acts as a γ-globin gene repressor also lays in a fact that *BCL11A* expression levels are much higher in adult compered to fetal developmental stage [54, 55]. As a direct repressor of fetal globin genes, BCL11A is the first genetically and biochemically validated regulator of the fetal to adult globin switch in humans [42] and, as such, represents potential target protein for HbF induction. However, since BCL11A acts as a transcriptional factor in non erythroid cells as well, recent studies have proposed GWAS-identified erythroid *BCL11A* enhancers as a particularly promising target for gene therapy in the β-thalassemia syndromes. This way, disruption of the *BCL11A* enhancers would only affect *BCL11A* expression in erythroid cells, while this gene expression would be intact in the non erythroid cells [56].

Genome-wide association studies indicate that variants in the *HBB*, *HSB1L- MYB* and *BCL11A* loci account for approximately 50% of the HbF level variation, suggesting that additional factors are involved [38, 39, 43, 57]. These factors may involve regulators of β-globin genes' expression (KLF1), proteins responsible for α-globin chain stability (AHSP) or factors involved in epigenetic regulation of fetal globin gene expression (FoP).

3.2.3. *KLF1 gene*

Erythroid Krüppel-like factor, (KLF1), previously known as EKLF, is one of the key erythroid-specific transcriptional factor that interacts with the CACCC box, important regulatory element of many erythroid genes, including adult β-globin gene and *BCL11A* [58, 59]. This interaction is carried out via three zinc finger domains, necessary for binding and activation of KLF1 target genes. KLF1 also contains proline-rich transactivation domain tough which this transcriptional factor preferentially activates the *HBB* gene at the expense of *HBG1/HBG2* gene expression by interacting directly with regulatory elements in *HBB* promoter [60-62]. Proline-rich region contains functionally distinct activation (AA 20-124) and inhibitory domains (AA 195-291). The minimal activation domain (AA 20-124) can be further divided into a subregion (AA 20-60) that itself does not activate, but interacts trough intermolecular interactions with another cellular protein, providing optimal transactivation potential to its adjacent (AA 60-124) sequence. At the same time, the inhibitory domain (AA 195-291) operates intramolecularly, preventing efficient binding of the DNA-binding zinc finger region within the same molecule [63]. Mutations affecting any of these functions of the KLF1 transcriptional factor, could potentially, directly or indirectly, alter expression of β-globin genes.

The direct association of mutations in human *KLF1* with hemoglobin regulation was first described by the Borg *et al.* [59], who reported a single point mutation in *KLF1* gene (p.K288X) responsible for completely abolishing the DNA binding domain resulting in KLF1 haploinsufficiency. Results from this study showed that this reduced KLF1 activity results in decreased *BCL11A* expression and hence, diminished synthesis of BCL11, γ-globin gene repressor. This, in turn, leads to increased HbF levels, observed in the carriers of p.K288X mutation [59, 64]. Similarly, novel *KLF1* mutation (c.914-4_914-1 del CTAG), hypothesized to affect splicing, causes haploinsufficiency of *KLF1*, leading to reduced expression levels of KLF1 target genes [65]. Results form our study on the first *KLF1* promoter mutation also go in favor of a KLF1 being a potent regulator of HbF levels [66]. Namely, results form this study suggest that this KLF1:g.-148G>A mutation leads to reduced *KLF1* gene transcription, which could explain, at least in part, the observed HPFH phenotype, further underlining the significant role of KLF1 on human fetal globin genes switching [66, 67].

Number of mutations affecting *KLF1* gene, as well as our understanding of different phenotypes associated with these mutations, are very obscure [68]. However, studies on *KLF1* gene mutations, including the ones without an obvious phenotype, contribute to the better understanding of the human erythropoiesis in general [59, 69-71].

3.2.4. AHSP gene

The αHb-stabilizing protein (AHSP), also known as erythroid-associated factor (ERAF), is erythroid-specific protein with an important role in erythropoiesis. Namely, it is involved in folding of the α-globin chains for β-globin association, heme binding, transfer for β-globin association and stabilization of α-globin chains. AHSP specifically binds multiple forms of α-globin including the apo form (no heme present) and α-hemoglobin (αHb) (α-globin with heme). Its role as a specific molecular chaperone that binds α-globin chain of hemoglobin preventing its precipitation, imply that alterations in *AHSP* gene expression or protein function could influence β-thalassemia phenotypes [72-74]. While some studies reported that reduced expression of *AHSP* was associated with a more severe phenotype among individuals with identical β-thalassemia and α-globin [75, 76], others indicated that AHSP is not a disease modifier of β-thalassemia [77, 78]. Research on *AHSP* gene mutation showed that structural mutations are uncommon, and therefore, not likely to be major modifiers of β-thalassemia. However, it remains a possibility that rare *AHSP* null or missense mutations, genetic or epigenetic factors unlinked to the gene, could modulate coexisting β-thalassemia [73, 77].

3.2.5. FoP protein

Friend of Prmt1 (FoP) is a small arginine/glycine rich protein encoded by the *C1orf77* gene. This protein, through its association with protein arginine methyltransferase 1 (PRMT1), is involved in transcriptional regulation of globin genes via histone methylation [79]. Studies have shown that this protein is a critical modulator of HbF levels, since knockdown of this factor leads to elevated γ-globin gene expression. Although it is unclear how FoP regulates γ-globin gene expression, it is presumed that this induction of fetal globin genes occurs trough modulation of SOX6 which acts as BCL11A cofactor, and not trough BCL11A itself. These results identify FoP as a novel potential therapeutic target in β-thalassemia syndromes, as well as in other hemoglobin-related disorders [80].

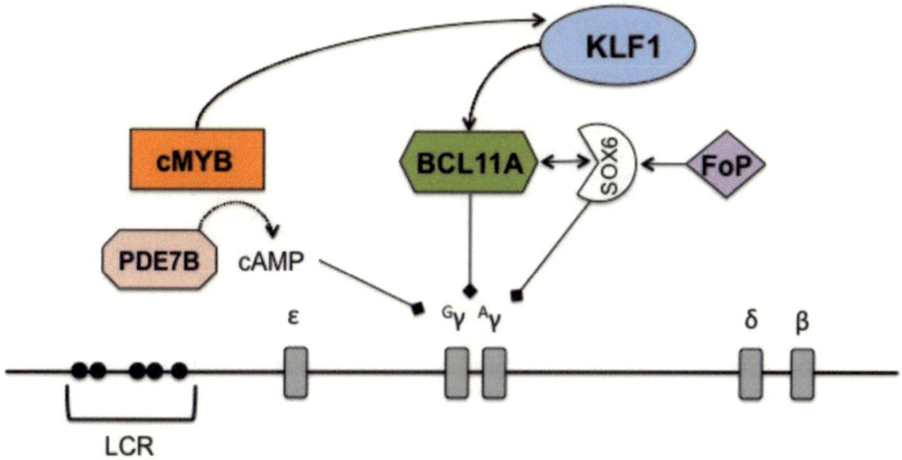

Figure 2. γ-globin gene regulators as potential targets for therapeutic induction of HbF. Human β-globin gene locus showing embryonic, fetal and adult globin genes, controlled by LCR. Transcription factors involved in regulation of γ-globin genes are shown. A line with an arrow at the end denotes positive regulation (activation). A line with a black box at the end denotes negative regulation (repression). Dashed line denotes ambiguous interaction. A line with arrows at two end points denotes mutual interaction. For details see the text.

4. Gene therapy

Despite immense achievement in the traditional care and treatment of β-thalassemia, including transfusion and drug therapy, until recently, a definitive cure for these disorders could only be achieved by bone marrow transplantation (BMT) from related or unrelated donors. However, BMT is available for only a small fraction of β-thalassemia patients and is characterized by relatively high mortality and morbidity, especially in the case of unrelated donors [27]. As an answer to these limitations of BMT and the need for more permanent solution, arose transfer of a therapeutic gene using autologous hematopoietic stem cells (HSC) as potential definitive cure for β-thalassemia syndromes.

The goal of this gene therapy is substitution of a defective or missing protein by introducing an intact copy of the faulty gene in question or by introduction of a gene which modifies the effect defected gene has on a cell such as β-thalassemia gene modifiers do.

For the successful gene therapy for β-hemoglobinopathies, several requirements need to be met. Those include high-efficiency gene transfer and high HSC engraftment; consistent levels of β-globin gene expression, independent of the site of integration; high expression levels of β-globin or γ-globin genes; regulated expression in the erythroid lineage; safe expression with little or no risk of insercional mutagenesis/oncogenesis [81].

Hematopoietic stem cells, as the targets for gene transfer, are harvested from patient bone marrow or peripheral blood following cytokine mobilization, purified by immunoselection, transduced and returned to the patient. Various types of vectors have been considered for gene transfer, including viral and non viral vectors [82].

4.1. Non viral vectors

Indication that gene therapy, as a therapy of the future for thalassemia syndromes, could be possible, came from the study on suppressor tRNA [83]. In this study a human tRNALys gene was converted to an amber suppressor by site-specific mutagenesis of the anticodon. As a result, a tRNA that suppressed the UAG amber nonsense mutation in β^0-thalassemia mRNA was produced giving rise to functional β-globin polypeptide. Although promising, the use of such genes in gene therapy would be limited to β^0-thalassemias due to nonsense mutations. Also, amber suppressor tRNA could suppress termination of the proteins with UAG as their normal termination codon making these genes not an ideal candidate for use in gene therapy.

As a potential approach to gene therapy for hemoglobin disorders, the catalytic properties of ribozymes to alter the defective mRNA produced by the mutated β-globin gene was also explored [84]. Namely, *trans*-acting group 1 ribozyme was created in a such a way that it was able to convert mutated β-globin transcript into RNA encoding γ-globin. This way, not only would the mutated gene be removed but it would be replaced with gene producing fetal globin chain. Although these results were very promising, several problems emerged, one of which is long-term effect of the therapy since it is directed at transcription product and not at the mutated gene itself [85].

Contrary to these non viral vectors, viral vectors showed higher gene transfer efficiency, since they do not require harsh physical means, such as electroporation, to enter the cell [86].

4.2. Viral vectors

The first viral vectors used to transfer the human β-globin gene in the mouse HSCs were oncoretroviruses or gamma-retroviruses (γRV), which efficiently transfer therapeutic gene into HSCs without transferring any viral genes. Gamma-retroviruses belong to the family of Retroviridae, which, among others, also include lentivirus (LV) and foamy virus (FV), both used in clinical trials or preclinical testing. These viral vectors are constructed in such a way that the genetic elements needed for pathogenicity and replication are removed and are replaced with the cellular transgene of interest [86, 87].

4.2.1. Retroviral vectors

The γRV vectors contain intact viral long terminal repeats (LTRs) which enclose U3, R and U5 regions. The U3 region has strong promoter and enhancer activity and is usually used by the virus to reverse transcribe and incorporate the genetic material into the host genome (Figure 3.) [86]. Early attempts to transfer human β-globin gene in the mouse HSCs using these vectors, resulted in tissue-specific, but low and variable human β-globin expression in bone marrow chimeras, usually varying between 0% and 2% of endogenous mouse β-globin mRNA levels [88]. In order to increase expression levels of transferred β-globin genes, efforts were made to include LCR elements of the β-globin gene locus into these γRV vectors. Incorporation of the LCR's DNase I hypersensitivity sites, HS2, HS3 and HS4, significantly increased expression levels in the murine erythroleukemia (MEL) cells, but failed to abolish positional variability expression and resulted in vectors with low titers [81, 87]. Gamma-retroviral vectors were also limited by their size, need for cell division before integration, as well as their stable transmission since they were so unstable that the transduced globin gene was very rarely integrated intact into the genome, thus losing any therapeutic efficacy [27].

4.2.2. Lentiviral vectors

Bioengineering of HIV-1 devoid of any pathogenic elements resulted in the development of lentiviral (LV) vectors as suitable vectors for high-efficiency gene transfer. In order to improve its safety, self-inactivating (SIN) LV vector was constructed by deleting the viral promoter/ enhancer in the U3 region of the 3′ LTR, without significant loss in titers or infectivity. During reverse transcription of the viral RNA, this deletion that gets copied to the 5′ LTR, minimizing transactivation of neighboring cellular promoters, thus improving the safety of the vector itself [89]. Instead of U3 region in the 5′ LTR, SIN LV vector contains a cytomegalovirus (CMV) promoter which is only used in packaging the vector and is not transmitted to the host cell (Figure 3.). This new generation of LV vectors display variety of advantages compared to γRV vectors including the ability to infect quiescent, nondividing long-term HSC (HSC capable of self renewal). Unlike γ RV vectors, SIN LV can stably carry larger and more complex transgene cassettes containing introns and regulatory elements, necessary for high globin gene expression. LV vectors usually insert these cassettes within gene introns, avoiding promoters and 5′ regulator regions which RV vectors have high affinity for [86, 90].

With the discovery of LV vectors as a potent transporter of gene of interest, research turned to the globin cassette itself. The first study to demonstrate stable transmission and high-level β-globin gene expression in a mouse model of β-thalassemia intermedia, tested two types of LV vectors. Larger, TNS9 vector, contained large LCR fragments encompassing HS2, HS3 and HS4 and was approximately 3.2 kb in size, while smaller, RNS1 vector carried only a minimal core LCR elements. It was shown that cells transduced with TNS9 vector sustained higher human β-globin transcript levels. Also, this vector achieved significant improvement in the hematocrits, red blood cell and reticulocyte count, as well as hemoglobin levels in β-thalassemia mice [91]. Today, vectors' globin cassette usually contains β-globin gene with deleted destabilizing Rsal fragment located within intron 2 and several sequences surrounding HS of the LCR. However, the number and the length of the HS sites vary in all globin cassettes, since

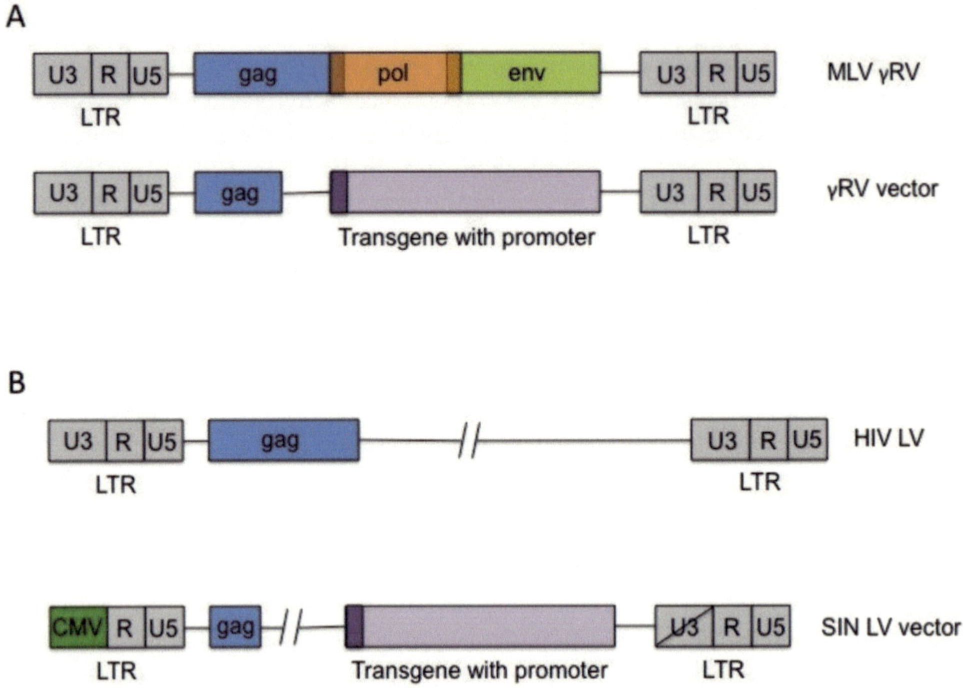

For details see the text.

Figure 3. A. Genome organization of MLV γRV and γRV vector; B. Genome organization of HIV LV and SIN LV vector.

it's proven very difficult to define really important regulatory sequence within each HS, while omitting potentially destabilizing elements. Also, some of the vectors in use are flanked by insulators, genomic element that can shelter genes from their surrounding chromosomal environment, resulting in position-independent expression [27].

5. Gene therapy ofβ -thalassemia: Success or fail?

The first successful human gene therapy for β-thalassemia was achieved in 2007., when HbE/ β^0-thalassemia major patient was transduced with vector containing antisickling β-globin (βA(T87Q)), a 260 bp long globin promoter, HS2, HS3, HS4 and two copies of insulator flanking the globin cassette. Although the patient became totally transfusion independent, it was discovered a dominant cell clone with integration site into the *HMGA2* gene, a potential oncogene. While it was shown that overexpression of *HMGA2* is mainly associated with benign tumors, this observation points out some of the limitation of lentiviral vector gene transfer, which include the need for improved efficiency of gene delivery and insertion of the gene into non-oncogenic sites [92].

As the secondary modifier genes begin to take a center stage in the fight against β-thalassemia syndromes, researchers turned to these genes as potential target genes in gene therapy for β-thalassemia. Namely, transduction of CD34 cells with lentiviral vector carrying a short hairpin RNA (shRNA) targeting the γ-globin gene repressor BCL11A, led to significant increase of HbF in differentiated erythroblasts, around 10% in cells derived from normal donors and from 33% to 45% in β-thalassemic cells [93].

In the past few years, induced pluripotent stem cells (iPSCs) emerged as an interesting candidate for gene transfer. iPSCs are generated from mature somatic cells derived from skin fibroblasts, amniotic fluid or chorionic villus of β-thalassemia patients, by transduction with number of specific transcriptional factors. More specifically, it was shown that fibroblasts derived from tail-tip of a mouse, homozygote for human sickle cell allele (β^S/β^S), and infected with retroviruses encoding for Oct4, Sox2, and Klf4 factors, as well as with a lentivirus encoding a 2-lox c-Myc cDNA, were transformed into iPSC. These iPS cells, after being infected with an adenovirus encoding Cre-recombinase to delete the lentivirus-transduced c-Myc copies, in order to reduce the potential risk of tumor formation due to c-Myc transgene expression, stained positive for pluripotency markers. They also had a normal karyotype, and generated teratomas and chimeras. iPSC obtained in such a way were later successfully used in specific correction of the sickle cell allele, by being electroporated with a construct containing the human wild type β-globin gene. [94].

iPSCs are easily obtainable and represent an endless source of stem cells for gene manipulation and correction strategies. Therefore, the major advantage of these cells, when it comes to gene therapy, is the possibility to screen and choose the ideal clone with safe integration and high transgene expression profile. Unfortunately, several obstacles stand in the way of iPSCs being successfully used in gene therapy, one of which is elimination of the transcriptional factors used for induction, once they are no longer needed. More importantly, it is necessary to establish the correct re-programming so that the iPSCs do not develop tumors [27, 86, 87].

6. Conclusion

The β-thalassemias are the best understood disorders at the molecular level. Accordingly, therapy protocols based on molecular basis of β-thalassemia have been designed as an example of novel approaches in disease treatment. However, there is no well established gene therapy protocol for β-thalassemia to date. Why is so difficult to design an appropriate "therapeutic gene", even for this monogenic disorder, and to deliver it to hematopoietic stem cells to achieve therapeutic effect in β-thalassemia patients? Despite extensive research, modern science does not understand a complex gene expression regulation of globin genes yet. First of all, there is very specific regulation of expression of globin genes during ontogenesis. Also, tissue (erythroid)-specific regulation is present. Moreover, globin genes are regulated in a cell-specific manner since they are expressed only in the certain stages during differentiation of erythroid cell lineage. Finally, there is coordination between expression of α- and β-globin genes.

Besides all that, our knowledge is accumulating, and there is no doubt that gene manipulation will begin to cure in near future. Certainly, only somatic gene therapy is considered, since germ-line gene therapy raises many unique ethical concerns. Hopefully, thanks to gene therapy, a large number of people suffering from β-thalassemia will have a long and better life, despite the predispositions. That way, an old proverb will finally become true: "Fato prudentia maior est" (Wisdom is stronger than destiny).

Acknowledgements

This work was supported by Ministry of Education, Science and Technological Development, Republic of Serbia (Grant No. III41004).

Author details

Sonja Pavlovic*, Milena Ugrin and Maja Stojiljkovic

*Address all correspondence to: sonya@sezampro.rs

Institute of Molecular Genetics and Genetic Engineering, University of Belgrade, Belgrade, Serbia

References

[1] Urosevic J, Djureinovic T, Poznanic J, Cvorkov-Drazic M, Bunjevacki G, Janic D, et al. Homogeneity of the Hb Lepore gene in FR Yugoslavia. Balkan Journal of Medical Genetic. 2001;4(1&2):29-32.

[2] Pavlovic S, Kuzmanovic M, Urosevic J, Poznanic J, Zoranovic T, Djordjevic V, et al. Severe central nervous system thrombotic events in hemoglobin Sabine patient. Eur J Haematol. 2004;72(1):67-70.

[3] Cao A, Galanello R. Beta-thalassemia. Genet Med. 2010;12(2):61-76.

[4] Forget BG. The Thalassemia Syndromes. In: Hoffman R, Benz Jr EJ, Shattil SJ, Furie B, Cohen HJ, Silberstin LE, et al., editors. Hematology basic principles and practice. Philadelphia, USA: Churchill Livngstone; 2000.

[5] Tangvarasittichai S. Thalassemia Syndrome. In: Ikehara K. (ed.) Advances in the Study of Genetic Disorders. Rijeka: InTech; 2011. Available from http://www.intechopen.com/books/advances-in-the-study-of-genetic-disorders/thalassemia-syndrome.

[6] Thein SL. Genetic insights into the clinical diversity of beta thalassaemia. Br J Haematol. 2004;124(3):264-74.

[7] Thein SL. Beta-thalassaemia. Baillieres Clin Haematol. 1998;11(1):91-126.

[8] Patrinos GP, de Krom M, de Boer E, Langeveld A, Imam AM, Strouboulis J, et al. Multiple interactions between regulatory regions are required to stabilize an active chromatin hub. Genes Dev. 2004;18(12):1495-509.

[9] Forget BG. Progress in understanding the hemoglobin switch. N Engl J Med. 2011;365(9):852-4.

[10] Sankaran VG, Orkin SH. The switch from fetal to adult hemoglobin. Cold Spring Harb Perspect Med. 2013;3(1):a011643.

[11] Hardison RC, Chui DH, Giardine B, Riemer C, Patrinos GP, Anagnou N, et al. HbVar: A relational database of human hemoglobin variants and thalassemia mutations at the globin gene server. Hum Mutat. 2002;19(3):225-33.

[12] Rund D, Rachmilewitz E. Beta-thalassemia. N Engl J Med. 2005;353(11):1135-46.

[13] Lettre G. The search for genetic modifiers of disease severity in the β-hemoglobinopathies. Cold Spring Harb Perspect Med. 2012;2(10).

[14] Kazazian HH. The thalassemia syndromes: molecular basis and prenatal diagnosis in 1990. Semin Hematol. 1990;27(3):209-28.

[15] Thein SL. Genetic modifiers of beta-thalassemia. Haematologica. 2005;90(5):649-60.

[16] Galanello R, Piras S, Barella S, Leoni GB, Cipollina MD, Perseu L, et al. Cholelithiasis and Gilbert's syndrome in homozygous beta-thalassaemia. Br J Haematol. 2001;115(4):926-8.

[17] Thein SL. Genetic modifiers of the beta-haemoglobinopathies. Br J Haematol. 2008;141(3):357-66.

[18] Eldor A, Rachmilewitz EA. The hypercoagulable state in thalassemia. Blood. 2002;99(1):36-43.

[19] Brankovic-Sreckovic V, Milic Rasic V, Djordjevic V, Kuzmanovic M, Pavlovic S. Arterial ischemic stroke in a child with beta-thalassemia trait and methylentetrahydrofolate reductase mutation. J Child Neurol. 2007;22(2):208-10.

[20] Economou-Petersen E, Aessopos A, Kladi A, Flevari P, Karabatsos F, Fragodimitri C, et al. Apolipoprotein E epsilon4 allele as a genetic risk factor for left ventricular failure in homozygous beta-thalassemia. Blood. 1998;92(9):3455-9.

[21] Miyata M, Smith JD. Apolipoprotein E allele-specific antioxidant activity and effects on cytotoxicity by oxidative insults and beta-amyloid peptides. Nat Genet. 1996;14(1):55-61.

[22] Bernini LF, Harteveld CL. Alpha-thalassaemia. Baillieres Clin Haematol. 1998;11(1): 53-90.

[23] Galanello R, Cao A. Gene test review. Alpha-thalassemia. Genet Med. 2011;13(2): 83-8.

[24] Grosso M, Sessa R, Puzone S, Storino MR, Izzo P. Molecular basis of thalassemia. In: Silverberg D (ed.) Anemia. Rijeka: InTech; 2012. Available from http://www.intechopen.com/books/anemia/molecular-basis-of-thalassemia.

[25] Gilman JG, Huisman TH. DNA sequence variation associated with elevated fetal G gamma globin production. Blood. 1985;66(4):783-7.

[26] Thein SL. Pathophysiology of beta thalassemia--a guide to molecular therapies. Hematology Am Soc Hematol Educ Program. 2005:31-7.

[27] Cao A, Moi P, Galanello R. Recent advances in β-thalassemias. Pediatr Rep. 2011;3(2):e17.

[28] Huang XD, Yang XO, Huang RB, Zhang HY, Zhao HL, Zhao YJ, et al. A novel four base-pair deletion within the Agamma-GLOBin gene promoter associated with slight increase of Agamma expression in adult. Am J Hematol. 2000;63(1):16-9.

[29] Giardina P, Rivella S. Thalassemia syndromes. In: Hoffman R, Benz EJ, Silberstein LE, Heslop HE, Weitz JI, Anastasi J. (ed.) Hematology, basic principles. 6th edition. Philadelphia, USA: Elsevier; 2013.

[30] Sankaran VG, Xu J, Byron R, Greisman HA, Fisher C, Weatherall DJ, et al. A functional element necessary for fetal hemoglobin silencing. N Engl J Med. 2011;365(9): 807-14.

[31] Thein SL. Molecular control of fetal hemoglobin production and the implication for therapy. Hematology education for European Hematology Association. 2008;2(1): 186-93.

[32] Superti-Furga G, Barberis A, Schaffner G, Busslinger M. The -117 mutation in Greek HPFH affects the binding of three nuclear factors to the CCAAT region of the gamma-globin gene. EMBO J. 1988;7(10):3099-107.

[33] Langdon SD, Kaufman RE. Gamma-globin gene promoter elements required for interaction with globin enhancers. Blood. 1998;91(1):309-18.

[34] Sykes K, Kaufman R. A naturally occurring gamma globin gene mutation enhances SP1 binding activity. Mol Cell Biol. 1990;10(1):95-102.

[35] Fischer KD, Nowock J. The T----C substitution at -198 of the A gamma-globin gene associated with the British form of HPFH generates overlapping recognition sites for two DNA-binding proteins. Nucleic Acids Res. 1990;18(19):5685-93.

[36] Chen Z, Luo HY, Basran RK, Hsu TH, Mang DW, Nuntakarn L, et al. A T-to-G transversion at nucleotide -567 upstream of HBG2 in a GATA-1 binding motif is associated with elevated hemoglobin F. Mol Cell Biol. 2008;28(13):4386-93.

[37] Dover GJ, Smith KD, Chang YC, Purvis S, Mays A, Meyers DA, et al. Fetal hemoglobin levels in sickle cell disease and normal individuals are partially controlled by an X-linked gene located at Xp22.2. Blood. 1992;80(3):816-24.

[38] Thein SL, Menzel S, Peng X, Best S, Jiang J, Close J, et al. Intergenic variants of HBS1L-MYB are responsible for a major quantitative trait locus on chromosome 6q23 influencing fetal hemoglobin levels in adults. Proc Natl Acad Sci U S A. 2007;104(27): 11346-51.

[39] Uda M, Galanello R, Sanna S, Lettre G, Sankaran VG, Chen W, et al. Genome-wide association study shows BCL11A associated with persistent fetal hemoglobin and amelioration of the phenotype of beta-thalassemia. Proc Natl Acad Sci U S A. 2008;105(5):1620-5.

[40] Haj Khelil A, Morinière M, Laradi S, Khelif A, Perrin P, Ben Chibani J, et al. Xmn I polymorphism associated with concomitant activation of Gγ and Aγ globin gene transcription on a β0-thalassemia chromosome. Blood Cells Mol Dis. 2011;46(2):133-8.

[41] Labie D, Dunda-Belkhodja O, Rouabhi F, Pagnier J, Ragusa A, Nagel RL. The -158 site 5' to the G gamma gene and G gamma expression. Blood. 1985;66(6):1463-5.

[42] Sankaran VG, Lettre G, Orkin SH, Hirschhorn JN. Modifier genes in Mendelian disorders: the example of hemoglobin disorders. Ann N Y Acad Sci. 2010;1214:47-56.

[43] Lettre G, Sankaran VG, Bezerra MA, Araújo AS, Uda M, Sanna S, et al. DNA polymorphisms at the BCL11A, HBS1L-MYB, and beta-globin loci associate with fetal hemoglobin levels and pain crises in sickle cell disease. Proc Natl Acad Sci U S A. 2008;105(33):11869-74.

[44] Wahlberg K, Jiang J, Rooks H, Jawaid K, Matsuda F, Yamaguchi M, et al. The HBS1L-MYB intergenic interval associated with elevated HbF levels shows characteristics of a distal regulatory region in erythroid cells. Blood. 2009;114(6):1254-62.

[45] Wilber A, Nienhuis AW, Persons DA. Transcriptional regulation of fetal to adult hemoglobin switching: new therapeutic opportunities. Blood. 2011;117(15):3945-53.

[46] Sankaran VG, Menne TF, Šćepanović D, Vergilio JA, Ji P, Kim J, et al. MicroRNA-15a and -16-1 act via MYB to elevate fetal hemoglobin expression in human trisomy 13. Proc Natl Acad Sci U S A. 2011;108(4):1519-24.

[47] Stadhouders R, Aktuna S, Thongjuea S, Aghajanirefah A, Pourfarzad F, van Ijcken W, et al. HBS1L-MYB intergenic variants modulate fetal hemoglobin via long-range MYB enhancers. J Clin Invest. 2014;124(4):1699-710.

[48] Wyszynski DF, Baldwin CT, Cleves MA, Amirault Y, Nolan VG, Farrell JJ, et al. Polymorphisms near a chromosome 6q QTL area are associated with modulation of fetal

hemoglobin levels in sickle cell anemia. Cell Mol Biol (Noisy-le-grand). 2004;50(1): 23-33.

[49] Tafrali C, Paizi A, Borg J, Radmilovic M, Bartsakoulia M, Giannopoulou E, et al. Genomic variation in the MAP3K5 gene is associated with β-thalassemia disease severity and hydroxyurea treatment efficacy. Pharmacogenomics. 2013;14(5):469-83.

[50] Bailey L, Kuroyanagi Y, Franco-Penteado CF, Conran N, Costa FF, Ausenda S, et al. Expression of the gamma-globin gene is sustained by the cAMP-dependent pathway in beta-thalassaemia. Br J Haematol. 2007;138(3):382-95.

[51] Chen Z, Luo HY, Steinberg MH, Chui DH. BCL11A represses HBG transcription in K562 cells. Blood Cells Mol Dis. 2009;42(2):144-9.

[52] Sankaran VG, Menne TF, Xu J, Akie TE, Lettre G, Van Handel B, et al. Human fetal hemoglobin expression is regulated by the developmental stage-specific repressor BCL11A. Science. 2008;322(5909):1839-42.

[53] Chakalova L, Osborne CS, Dai YF, Goyenechea B, Metaxotou-Mavromati A, Kattamis A, et al. The Corfu deltabeta thalassemia deletion disrupts gamma-globin gene silencing and reveals post-transcriptional regulation of HbF expression. Blood. 2005;105(5):2154-60.

[54] Bauer DE, Orkin SH. Update on fetal hemoglobin gene regulation in hemoglobinopathies. Curr Opin Pediatr. 2011;23(1):1-8.

[55] Sankaran VG, Xu J, Orkin SH. Transcriptional silencing of fetal hemoglobin by BCL11A. Ann N Y Acad Sci. 2010;1202:64-8.

[56] Bauer DE, Kamran SC, Lessard S, Xu J, Fujiwara Y, Lin C, et al. An erythroid enhancer of BCL11A subject to genetic variation determines fetal hemoglobin level. Science. 2013;342(6155):253-7.

[57] Thein SL, Menzel S, Lathrop M, Garner C. Control of fetal hemoglobin: new insights emerging from genomics and clinical implications. Hum Mol Genet. 2009;18(R2):R216-23.

[58] Chen X, Reitman M, Bieker JJ. Chromatin structure and transcriptional control elements of the erythroid Krüppel-like factor (EKLF) gene. J Biol Chem. 1998;273(39): 25031-40.

[59] Borg J, Papadopoulos P, Georgitsi M, Gutiérrez L, Grech G, Fanis P, et al. Haploinsufficiency for the erythroid transcription factor KLF1 causes hereditary persistence of fetal hemoglobin. Nat Genet. 2010;42(9):801-5.

[60] Ouyang L, Chen X, Bieker JJ. Regulation of erythroid Krüppel-like factor (EKLF) transcriptional activity by phosphorylation of a protein kinase casein kinase II site within its interaction domain. J Biol Chem. 1998;273(36):23019-25.

[61] Donze D, Townes TM, Bieker JJ. Role of erythroid Kruppel-like factor in human gamma- to beta-globin gene switching. J Biol Chem. 1995;270(4):1955-9.

[62] Zhou D, Pawlik KM, Ren J, Sun CW, Townes TM. Differential binding of erythroid Krupple-like factor to embryonic/fetal globin gene promoters during development. J Biol Chem. 2006;281(23):16052-7.

[63] Chen X, Bieker JJ. Erythroid Krüppel-like factor (EKLF) contains a multifunctional transcriptional activation domain important for inter- and intramolecular interactions. EMBO J. 1996;15(21):5888-96.

[64] Zhou D, Liu K, Sun CW, Pawlik KM, Townes TM. KLF1 regulates BCL11A expression and gamma- to beta-globin gene switching. Nat Genet. 2010;42(9):742-4.

[65] Gallienne AE, Dréau HM, Schuh A, Old JM, Henderson S. Ten novel mutations in the erythroid transcription factor KLF1 gene associated with increased fetal hemoglobin levels in adults. Haematologica. 2012;97(3):340-3.

[66] Radmilovic M, Zukic B, Petrovic MS, Bartsakoulia M, Stankovic B, Kotur N, et al. Functional analysis of a novel KLF1 gene promoter variation associated with hereditary persistence of fetal hemoglobin. Ann Hematol. 2013;92(1):53-8.

[67] Tallack MR, Perkins AC. Three fingers on the switch: Krüppel-like factor 1 regulation of γ-globin to β-globin gene switching. Curr Opin Hematol. 2013;20(3):193-200.

[68] Borg J, Patrinos GP, Felice AE, Philipsen S. Erythroid phenotypes associated with KLF1 mutations. Haematologica. 2011;96(5):635-8.

[69] Satta S, Perseu L, Moi P, Asunis I, Cabriolu A, Maccioni L, et al. Compound heterozygosity for KLF1 mutations associated with remarkable increase of fetal hemoglobin and red cell protoporphyrin. Haematologica. 2011;96(5):767-70.

[70] Arnaud L, Saison C, Helias V, Lucien N, Steschenko D, Giarratana MC, et al. A dominant mutation in the gene encoding the erythroid transcription factor KLF1 causes a congenital dyserythropoietic anemia. Am J Hum Genet. 2010;87(5):721-7.

[71] Giardine B, Borg J, Higgs DR, Peterson KR, Philipsen S, Maglott D, et al. Systematic documentation and analysis of human genetic variation in hemoglobinopathies using the microattribution approach. Nat Genet. 2011;43(4):295-301.

[72] George E, Ann TJ. Genotype-phenotype diversity of beta-thalassemia in Malaysia: treatment options and emerging therapies. Med J Malaysia. 2010;65(4):256-60.

[73] dos Santos CO, Zhou S, Secolin R, Wang X, Cunha AF, Higgs DR, et al. Population analysis of the alpha hemoglobin stabilizing protein (AHSP) gene identifies sequence variants that alter expression and function. Am J Hematol. 2008;83(2):103-8.

[74] Bank A. AHSP: a novel hemoglobin helper. J Clin Invest. 2007;117(7):1746-9.

[75] Lai MI, Jiang J, Silver N, Best S, Menzel S, Mijovic A, et al. Alpha-haemoglobin stabilising protein is a quantitative trait gene that modifies the phenotype of beta-thalassaemia. Br J Haematol. 2006;133(6):675-82.

[76] Galanello R, Perseu L, Giagu N, Sole G. AHSP expression in beta-thalassemia carriers with thalassemia intermedia phenotype. Blood. 2003;102(1881a).

[77] Viprakasit V, Tanphaichitr VS, Chinchang W, Sangkla P, Weiss MJ, Higgs DR. Evaluation of alpha hemoglobin stabilizing protein (AHSP) as a genetic modifier in patients with beta thalassemia. Blood. 2004;103(9):3296-9.

[78] Wang Z, Yu W, Li Y, Shang X, Zhang X, Xiong F, et al. Analysis of alpha-hemoglobin-stabilizing protein (AHSP) gene as a genetic modifier to the phenotype of beta-thalassemia in Southern China. Blood Cells Mol Dis. 2010;45(2):128-32.

[79] Ginder GD. Epigenetic regulation of fetal globin gene expression in adult erythroid cells. Transl Res. 2015;165(1):115-25.

[80] van Dijk TB, Gillemans N, Pourfarzad F, van Lom K, von Lindern M, Grosveld F, et al. Fetal globin expression is regulated by Friend of Prmt1. Blood. 2010;116(20): 4349-52.

[81] Arumugam P, Malik P. Genetic therapy for beta-thalassemia: from the bench to the bedside. Hematology Am Soc Hematol Educ Program. 2010;2010:445-50.

[82] Nienhuis AW, Persons DA. Development of gene therapy for thalassemia. Cold Spring Harb Perspect Med. 2012;2(11).

[83] Temple GF, Dozy AM, Roy KL, Kan YW. Construction of a functional human suppressor tRNA gene: an approach to gene therapy for beta-thalassaemia. Nature. 1982;296(5857):537-40.

[84] Lan N, Howrey RP, Lee SW, Smith CA, Sullenger BA. Ribozyme-mediated repair of sickle beta-globin mRNAs in erythrocyte precursors. Science. 1998;280(5369):1593-6.

[85] Weatherall DJ. Gene therapy: repairing haemoglobin disorders with ribozymes. Curr Biol. 1998;8(19):R696-8.

[86] Chandrakasan S, Malik P. Gene therapy for hemoglobinopathies: the state of the field and the future. Hematol Oncol Clin North Am. 2014;28(2):199-216.

[87] Raja JV, Rachchh MA, Gokani RH. Recent advances in gene therapy for thalassemia. J Pharm Bioallied Sci. 2012;4(3):194-201.

[88] Lisowski L, Sadelain M. Current status of globin gene therapy for the treatment of beta-thalassaemia. Br J Haematol. 2008;141(3):335-45.

[89] Malik P, Arumugam PI. Gene Therapy for beta-thalassemia. Hematology Am Soc Hematol Educ Program. 2005:45-50.

[90] Nienhuis AW. Development of gene therapy for blood disorders: an update. Blood. 2013;122(9):1556-64.

[91] May C, Rivella S, Callegari J, Heller G, Gaensler KM, Luzzatto L, et al. Therapeutic haemoglobin synthesis in beta-thalassaemic mice expressing lentivirus-encoded human beta-globin. Nature. 2000;406(6791):82-6.

[92] Cavazzana-Calvo M, Payen E, Negre O, Wang G, Hehir K, Fusil F, et al. Transfusion independence and HMGA2 activation after gene therapy of human β-thalassaemia. Nature. 2010;467(7313):318-22.

[93] Wilber A, Hargrove PW, Kim YS, Riberdy JM, Sankaran VG, Papanikolaou E, et al. Therapeutic levels of fetal hemoglobin in erythroid progeny of β-thalassemic CD34+ cells after lentiviral vector-mediated gene transfer. Blood. 2011;117(10):2817-26.

[94] Hanna J, Wernig M, Markoulaki S, Sun CW, Meissner A, Cassady JP, et al. Treatment of sickle cell anemia mouse model with iPS cells generated from autologous skin. Science. 2007;318(5858):1920-3.

Chapter 9

Sickle Cell Disease – Current Treatment and New Therapeutical Approaches

Thais Regina Ferreira de Melo,
Lucas dos Reis Ercolin, Rafael Consolin Chelucci,
Aylime Castanho Bolognesi Melchior,
Carolina Lanaro, Chung Man Chin and
Jean Leandro dos Santos

Additional information is available at the end of the chapter

http://dx.doi.org/10.5772/60515

Abstract

Sickle cell disease (SCD) is one of the most common genetic disorders worldwide. It is caused by a point mutation that changes glutamic acid (Glu6) to valine (Val6) in the β chain of hemoglobin. Vaso-occlusion is the most well-known problem associated with SCD. Despite recent advances in understanding the disease at the molecular level, few therapeutic strategies are available. Hydroxyurea is the only drug currently approved by the U.S. Food and Drug Administration for the disease, and it has serious adverse effects and lack of efficacy in some patients. However, new therapeutic approaches are under investigation in the hope of discovering new drugs to treat SCD. These include agents that: a) increase nitric oxide bioavailability; b) modify the rheological properties of the blood; c) bind covalently to hemoglobin; d) prevent hemoglobin dehydration; e) reduce iron overload; and f) induce the expression of gamma globin and fetal hemoglobin. In this chapter, we discuss the current treatment of SCD and the advances made in medicinal chemistry to find new drugs to treat this neglected hematological disease.

Keywords: Sickle cell disease, hemoglobinopathy, gamma globin, fetal hemoglobin, drug discovery

1. Introduction

1.1. General background

Sickle cell disease (SCD) is one of the most prevalent hemoglobinopathies worldwide. It has been hypothesized that this disease originated millions of years ago, in the sub-Saharan countries in mid-western Africa, eastern Asia, and some regions of India [1]. The distribution of the disease correlates with the malaria-endemic regions because it confers a protective effect against infection by the plasmodium [1-3].

Many biochemical and immunological mechanisms have been investigated to explain the protection conferred by hemoglobin S (HbS) against malaria. Infected sickle erythrocytes are known to be phagocytized faster than normal erythrocytes, thereby reducing parasitemia [4]; however, despite the many studies of the complex mechanisms involved, their relevance *in vivo* remains unclear [5].

According to the World Health Organization, about 5% of the world population carried a gene mutation for a hemoglobinopathy in 2011, particularly those mutations causing SCD and thalassemia. Today, SCD is not restricted to Africa and parts of India, but is found in the America and Europe, mainly as a result of migration and racial intermingling. In the United States, the disease afflicts approximately 1:500 Afro-American and 1:4000 Hispanic-American neonates [6].

The Brazilian National Program of Neonatal Screening estimates that around 2 million individuals carry the HbS trait in that country and 25,000–50,000 individuals are homozygous for HbS. About 3,500 children are thought to be born with SCD every year and 200,000 are heterozygous for the HbS gene [7-8].

1.2. Pathophysiology

Sickle cell disease is characterized by a point mutation in the sixth codon of the β-globin gene. The replacement of a thymine residue with an adenine (GTG to GAG) results in the substitution of glutamic acid for valine in the β-chain of hemoglobin, thus producing an anomalous hemoglobin (β^s-globin). After several cycles of deoxygenation and oxygenation, the HbS molecule polymerizes. This process is facilitated during the deoxygenation state of hemoglobin S (HbS) by hydrophobic interactions between the β subunits of the hemoglobin tetramer. The polymers thus formed can damage the erythrocyte structure, leading to sickle-shaped erythrocytes [9].

The polymerization of HbS represents the primary event in the molecular pathogenesis of the disease, and this process is dependent on several factors, including the concentrations of HbS and oxygen, the presence of high levels of normal hemoglobin, pH, temperature, and ionic strength [10]. HbS polymerization is responsible for: a) altering the structure and flexibility of the erythrocytes; b) promoting erythrocyte dehydration; and c) physical and oxidative stress [11, 12]. All of these events contribute to the hemolysis of the erythrocytes. The heme group present in the hemoglobin is then released into the circulation and can capture the nitric oxide

(NO) molecules present in the vascular endothelium, generating a "vasoconstriction effect" in the patient [13]. Low levels of NO contribute to the vasculopathy and hypercoagulability characteristic of the disease, and have been related to its clinical manifestations, including pulmonary hypertension, leg ulcers, priapism, and cerebrovascular disease [14, 15].

NO is an important mediator of cell functions, with various effects, including vasodilatation, the inhibition of platelet aggregation, and the reduced expression of adhesive molecules (Figure 1). This mediator also stimulates the expression of the gamma globin gene and consequently increases the production of fetal hemoglobin (HbF). This mechanism seems to involve soluble guanylyl cyclase (sGC), which increases the expression of γ-globin in erythroleukemic cells and primary erythroblasts [16, 17].

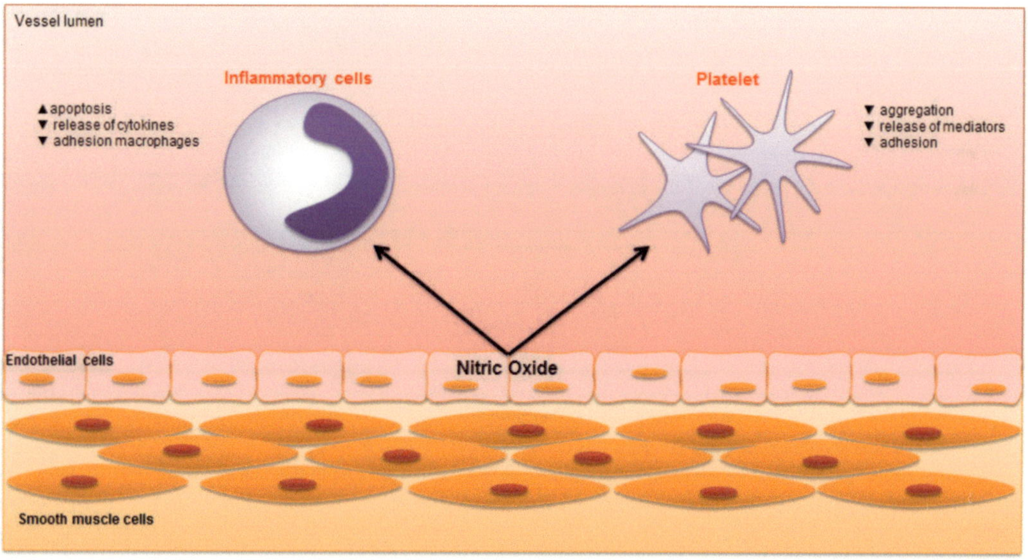

Figure 1. Effects of nitric oxide on the vascular endothelium, inflammatory cells, and platelets.

Another manifestation of SCD is vaso-occlusion (Figure 2), which is the major cause of morbidity in patients with SCD, causing tissue infarct, painful crises, acute thoracic syndrome, and nephropathy. The interactions of the sickle erythrocytes, leucocytes, neutrophils, and platelets with the vascular endothelium increase, leading to the formation of heterocellular aggregates, which are responsible for vaso-occlusion [18]. Mechanistically, the interaction between the erythrocytes and the endothelium involves $\alpha4\beta1$ integrin, expressed on the erythrocyte surface, and fibronectin, vascular cell adhesion protein 1 (VCAM-1), intracellular adhesion molecule 1 (ICAM-1), and E-selectin, expressed on the endothelial cell surface [19]. Other ligands, including thrombospondin, von Willebrand factor, immunoglobulins, and fibrinogen, also seem to contribute to this adherence [20].

This vaso-occlusion is aggravated by ischemic cycles, which cause oxidative and inflammatory stress and increase the production of proinflammatory cytokines [21, 22].

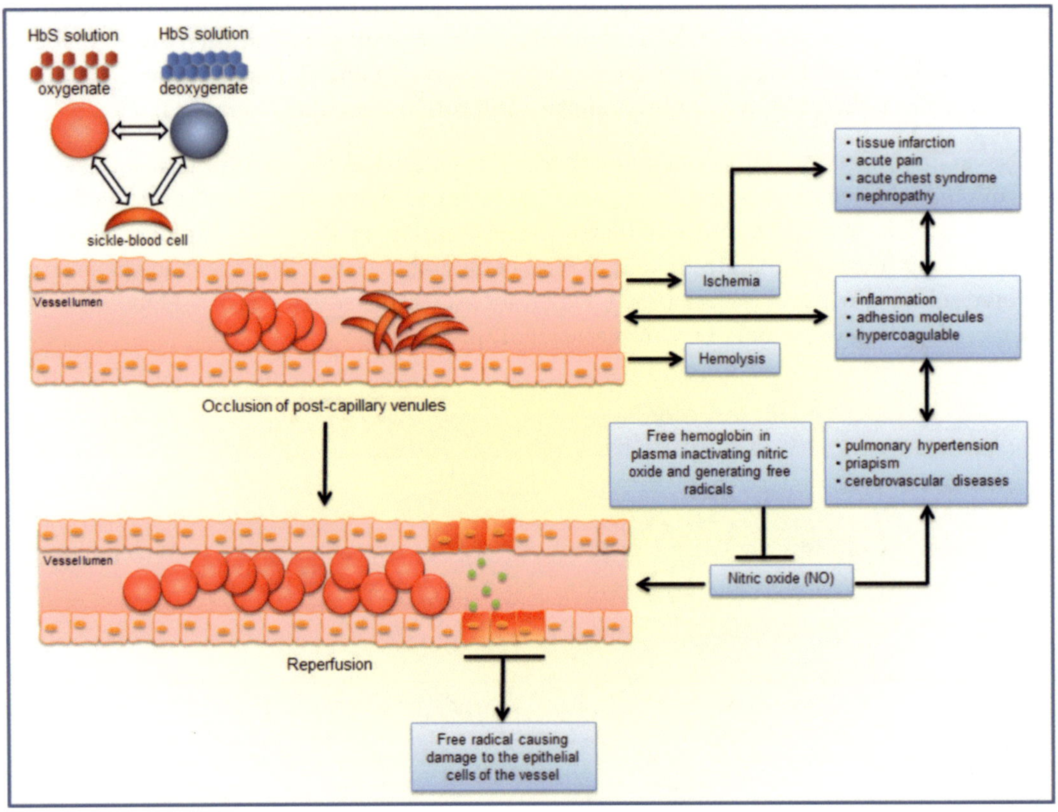

Figure 2. Pathophysiology of sickle cell disease.

Inflammation is another central feature of the vasculopathy of SCD (Figure 2). The adhesion and activation of leucocytes increase the production of proinflammatory cytokines, such as tumor necrosis factor α (TNF-α), interleukin 1β (IL-1β), and IL-8, which contribute to chronic inflammation and vaso-occlusive crises [23, 24]. SCD patients show increased levels of proinflammatory cytokines, including TNF-α [25], and high levels of TNF-α can increase the chemotactic proprieties of cells and amplify inflammation. This cytokine is also responsible for: a) increasing neutrophil adherence to the vascular endothelium; b) stimulating the production of free radicals; c) stimulating the synthesis of other inflammatory mediators, such as IL-1β and prostaglandin E2 (PGE_2); and d) modulating coagulation and anticoagulation functions [26, 27]. Therefore, the increased plasma levels of TNF-α in SCD patients contribute to their vaso-occlusive crises and inflammatory episodes [25, 28-29].

1.3. Treatment

Despite current advances in medical technology, there is still no specific treatment for SCD. The drugs available can only reduce the symptoms and increase the patient's quality of life. The complexity of SCD is an obstacle to the scientific development of new selective and effective therapies. This is coupled with the lack of interest within the pharmaceutical industry in searching for new drugs for this disease, another major impediment to the discovery of new treatments [30, 31]. Here, we discuss the main strategies and current advances in the search for new drugs with which to treat SCD.

Several strategies and therapies can be explored for the treatment of SCD. Among these, we include: a) the induction of HbF synthesis; b) the inhibition of erythrocyte dehydration; c) the inhibition of cellular adhesion; d) vasodilators; e) adenosine agonists; f) hemoglobin modifiers; g) Rho-kinase inhibition; and h) chelating agents (Figure 3). All of these strategies are discussed below.

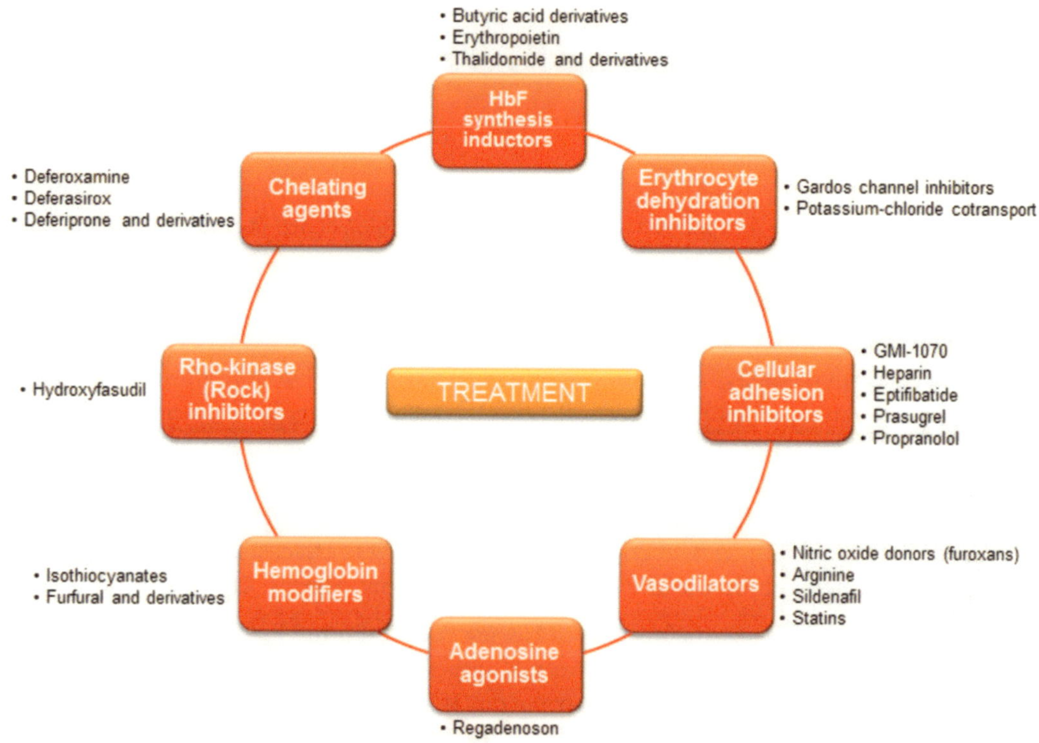

Figure 3. Therapeutic strategies for the treatment of SCD.

Induction of HbF synthesis

The induction of HbF synthesis is a promising strategy for the treatment of SCD [32, 33]. The elevated levels of HbS and low levels of HbF in patients with SCD are related to the clinical severity of the disease and the early mortality of the patients. This effect is related to high levels of HbS polymerization and its increased adherence to the vascular endothelium, which aggravate the vaso-occlusive process [34, 35]. Agents that increase HbF levels include hydroxyurea (HU), decitabine, azacitidine, NO donors, butyric acid and its derivatives, erythropoietin, and thalidomide and its derivatives.

• Hydroxyurea

Hydroxyurea (Figure 4) is a chemotherapeutic agent and selective inhibitor of ribonucleoside diphosphate reductase, an enzyme that converts ribonucleoside diphosphates to deoxyribonucleoside diphosphates. Therefore, HU inhibits the G1/S phase transition of the cell cycle [36]. Currently, it is the only drug approved by the U.S. Food and Drug Administration (FDA) for the treatment of SCD.

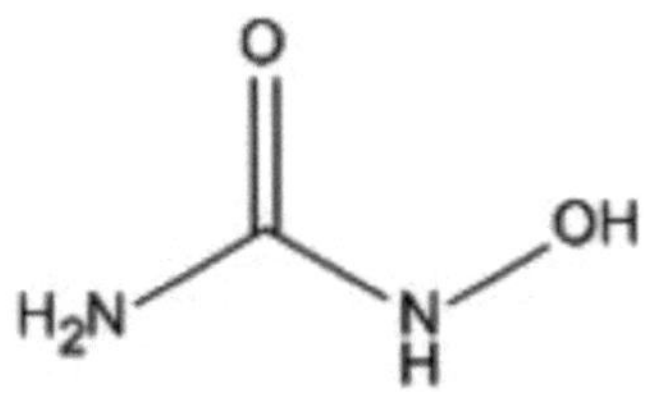

Figure 4. Chemical structure of hydroxyurea.

HU reduces the number of vaso-occlusive crises, episodes of acute thoracic syndrome, and urgent requirement for blood transfusion [37]. One nine-year clinical study demonstrated a reduction of 40% in the number of fatalities among patients treated with this drug [38].

The beneficial effects of HU in SCD are related to the increase of HbF levels. Some data suggest that the mechanism whereby HU increases the levels of HbF involves its biotransformation of NO, which activates the soluble guanylate cyclase (sGC) on erythroid cells [17, 39]. The activation of sGC increases the expression of γ-globin in erythroleukemic cells and primary human erythroblasts [16]. Other effects of HU include the reduction of leukocytes, reticulocytes, and platelets, and a reduction in the adhesiveness of erythrocytes and leukocytes to the vascular endothelium [40]. However, HU has several adverse effects, such as myelotoxicity, cutaneous hyperpigmentation, and ulcerative lesions on lower limbs [41].

Despite these adverse effects, the benefits of HU use are supported by evidence of its efficacy in reducing morbidity and mortality. However, importantly, about one third of patients do not respond to HU treatment [42]. In this context it is important to introduce new drugs that recapitulate the beneficial effects of HU without its potential toxicity.

• NO donors

Nitric oxide is a gas, synthetized from L-arginine by a family of enzymes called nitric oxide synthases [43], which have multiple regulatory functions in organisms, as transcription factor activators, in glycolysis and mitochondrial electron transport, hormone release, penile erection, and platelet and neutrophil adhesion, among others [44].

NO is the main endothelium-derived relaxant, with a central role in homeostasis and the inhibition of platelet aggregation [45]. It is also considered an epigenetic molecule because it bonds with the sulfhydryl groups of cysteine residues, generating S-nitrosyl groups, which can modify gene expression [46, 47]. The most important example of the modification of gene expression by NO involves the activity of histone deacetylase (HDAC2), in which cysteine residues 262 and 274 are S-nitrosylated, causing the enzyme to dissociate from the chromatin, resulting in acetylation of the H3 and H4 histones [48].

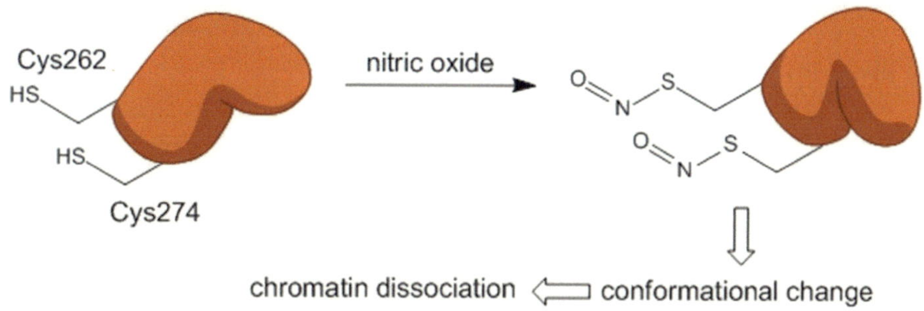

Figure 5. Representation of the NO effect on HDAC2 S-nitrosylation.

- Decitabine and azacitidine

Decitabine (5-aza-2′-deoxycytidine) (Figure 6) is a potent inducer of HbF synthesis, acting through the hypomethylation of the promoter of the γ-globin gene [49]. One clinical study conducted with a small group of patients showed that decitabine increases HbF production, even in patients unresponsive to HU [50]. In animal models, decitabine does not induce carcinogenesis and, curiously, has shown protective activity against cancer [51].

Azacitidine (5-azacytidine) (Figure 6) has also been shown to act as an inducer of HbF. However, serious adverse effects in humans and animals have restricted its use in the treatment of SCD, including carcinogenicity, neutropenia, thrombocytopenia, and leukopenia [52, 53].

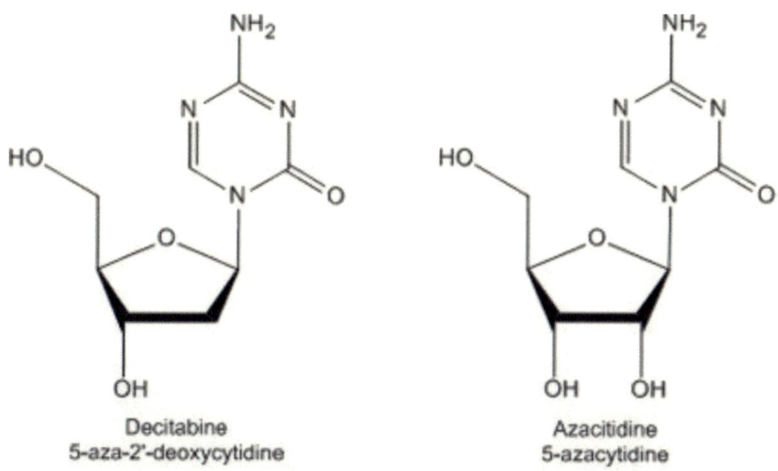

Figure 6. Chemical structure of decitabine and its analogue, azacitidine.

- Butyric acid and its derivatives

The butyrates (Figure 7) are short-chain fatty acids that inhibit the histone deacetylases, resulting in the induction of γ-globin gene expression and the synthesis of HbF [54]. The butyrates have been shown to produce a sustained increase in the HbF concentrations of SCD patients, but their short half-lives and low bioavailability have limited their use clinically. Therefore, new derivatives of butyric acid, with superior bioavailability and increased half-lives, are under investigation in animal models [33, 55].

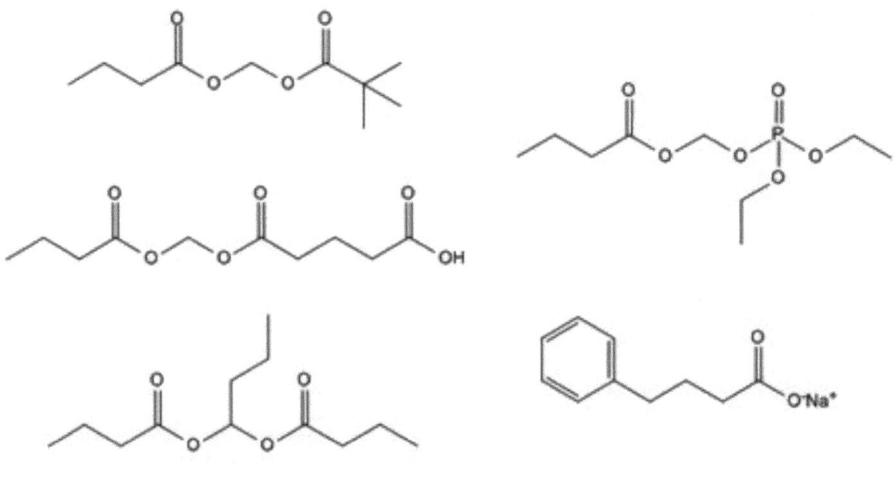

Figure 7. Chemical structures of some butyric acid derivatives.

- Erythropoietin

Recombinant human erythropoietin also increases HbF levels *in vivo* and *in vivo* with few adverse effects. This combination has shown good results, with a better tolerance profile than either agent alone, mainly in patients who are only weakly responsive to HU [56].

- Thalidomide and its derivatives

Thalidomide (Figure 8), originally used as a hypnotic/sedative and antiemetic agent, was withdrawn from the market in the 1960s because of its teratogenic effects [57]. However, it has proven useful in the treatment of other diseases, such as leprosy and multiple myeloma, based on its anti-inflammatory and immunomodulatory effects [58].

Thalidomide increases the production of reactive oxygen species (ROS) and induces γ-globin mRNA expression in a dose-dependent manner, *via* p38 MAPK signaling and histone H4 acetylation [59]. High levels of ROS act as signals that mediate the phosphorylation of tyrosine kinases, such as p38 MAPK, thereby regulating the expression of γ-globin [60].

Lenalidomide and pomalidomide (Figure 8) are thalidomide analogues with immunomodulatory effects related, in part, to the inhibition of TNF-α [61]. Moutouh-de Parseval et al. (2008) have shown that pomalidomide and lenalidomide induce HbF synthesis and modulate erythrocyte differentiation, and these effects were improved when the authors combined the treatment with HU. The combination of HU with pomalidomide was more effective that its combination with lenalidomide [62]. *In vivo* studies of these two agents in transgenic animals have shown increased HbF expression, without any myelosuppressive effect, at levels similar to those in the HU-treated controls [63].

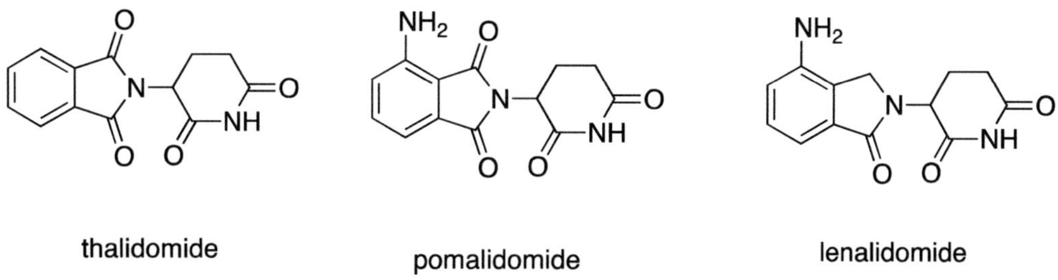

Figure 8. Chemical structures of thalidomide, pomalidomide and lenalidomide.

Inhibition of erythrocyte dehydration

HbS polymerization is dependent on the intracellular concentration of HbS, which is directly related to the hydration state of the cell. Therefore, strategies that prevent cellular dehydration should be explored for the treatment of SCD. The inhibition of potassium–chloride cotransport, in which potassium causes the movement of chloride ions and water, produces an osmotic imbalance and causes dehydration, with further polymerization of HbS [64]. The calcium-activated potassium channel known as the Gardos channel is also present on sickle erythrocytes and could be inhibited to promote an adequate osmotic balance [65]. Examples of compounds that inhibit this channel include magnesium, clotrimazole, and senicapoc.

- Magnesium

It has been reported that increased levels of intracellular Mg^{2+} inhibit the efflux of potassium from the erythrocyte, preventing its dehydration [66]. Preliminary studies in transgenic animals with SCD have shown that magnesium supplementation can substantially reduce the cotransport of KCl, and therefore reduce the mean corpuscular volume and the reticulocytes number [67]. Magnesium pidolate combined with HU was tested for six months in a clinical study (phase I) involving children. The results showed that magnesium pidolate reduces KCl cotransport activity. However, the authors found no changes in other hematological parameters [68].

- Clotrimazole

The antifungal drug clotrimazole (Figure 9) inhibits the Gardos channel in erythrocytes, but this drug is known for its adverse effects during long-term therapy [67].Despite its toxicity, clotrimazole was used as a prototype molecule for molecular modification, which has generated compounds such as NS3623 and xlink652, which inhibit the Gardos channel. These compounds prevented hemolysis and sickle cell formation *in vivo*, in a transgenic mouse model [69, 70].

- ICA-17043 (Senicapoc)

Preclinical studies using the compound ICA-17043 (Figure 9) have shown that it reduces the activity of the Gardos channel, thus reducing the hemoglobin concentration and hemolysis. However, despite these beneficial effects, no reduction in the frequency of vaso-occlusion episodes was observed [71].

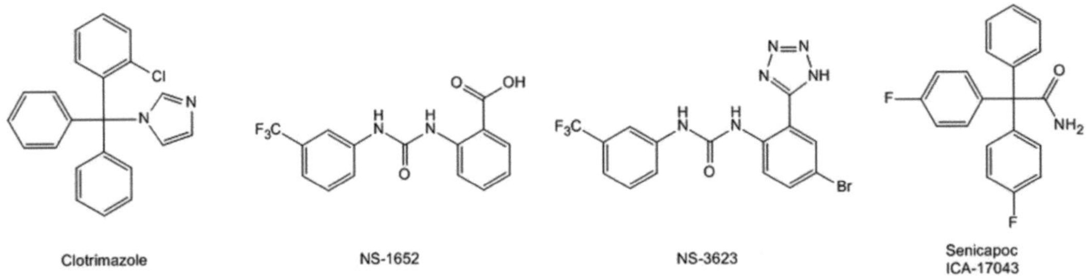

Figure 9. Chemical structures of erythrocyte dehydration inhibitors.

Inhibition of cellular adhesion

The adhesion of sickle cells to the vascular endothelium involves various mediators, including integrin $\alpha4\beta1$, CD36, and ICAM-4, which are responsible for the cellular interaction with the endothelium directly through E-selectin, P-selectin, integrins, and VCAM-1, or indirectly through molecules such as thrombospondin and von Willebrand factor [72, 73]. Several compounds have demonstrated a capacity to inhibit cellular adhesion, including rivipansel, heparin, eptifibatide, prasugrel, and propranolol.

Rivipansel (Figure 10), a synthetic glycomimetic molecule, is a pan-selectin inhibitor that acts on E-, P-, and L-selectin. It has been shown to restore blood flow during vaso-occlusion, increasing the survival rates in treated animals. An *in vivo* study indicated that this drug is a potent inhibitor of neutrophil adhesion through its interaction with E-selectin and ICAM-1 [74].

Heparin potentially interferes with the adhesion of sickle cells to the vascular endothelium through P-selectin. Clinical trials of low-molecular-weight heparin reported a reduction in the duration and severity of acute vaso-occlusive episodes [55, 73].

Another drug under investigation for the treatment of SCD is eptifibatide. Phase I clinical trials of eptifibatide, a synthetic cyclic peptide antagonist of glycoprotein IIb/IIIa (or integrin $\alpha_{IIb}\beta_3$), have reported reductions in platelet activation and inflammatory markers [75].

Vasodilators

Vasodilation is a desirable effect in the prevention of vaso-occlusive processes. NO is a vasodilator synthesized from L-arginine by endothelial cells and is responsible for maintaining vascular tonus [13]. It has been demonstrated that therapies that increase the bioavailability of NO may be beneficial to SCD patients, because 50% of patients showed endothelial dysfunction attributable to low endothelial levels of NO [76].

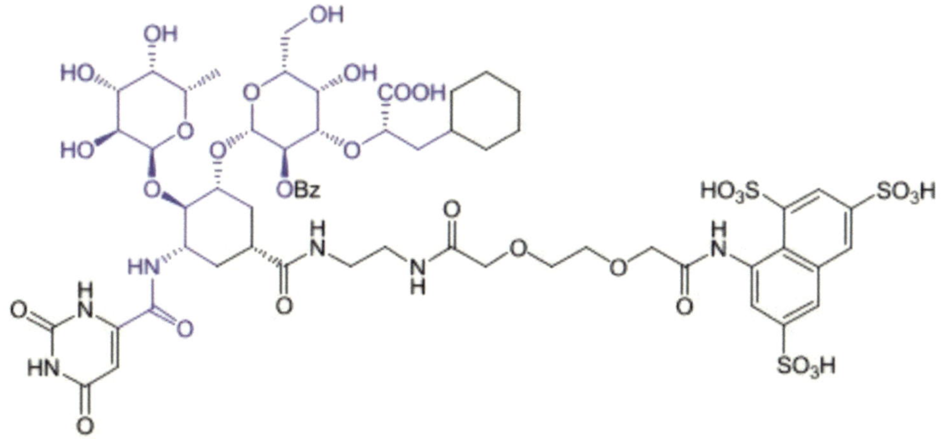

Figure 10. Chemical structure of rivipansel (GMI-1070).

NO is a soluble gas with a short half-life, used for pulmonary hypertension in newborn children. Its first use in SCD was reported by Atz and Wessel (1997), for the treatment of acute thoracic syndrome. NO inhalation reduces vascular pressure and resistance, and improves oxygenation in SCD patients [77]..

NO donors containing the organic nitrate ester subunit and furoxan derivatives have been evaluated as potential compounds with which to treat SCD. Santos et al (2011 and 2012) synthetized new hybrid compounds containing the thalidomide subunit, an organic nitrate ester, and furoxan derivatives, as NO donors (Figure 11). All the molecules have shown NO-donor ability, with anti-inflammatory and analgesic effects. The compounds also induced gamma globin expression and HbF synthesis *in vivo* [78, 79].

Arginine supplementation can also increase NO levels, especially in patients suffering vaso-occlusive events [80]. Arginine also reduces the pulmonary arterial pressure in patients with pulmonary hypertension [81].

Sildenafil is a phosphodiesterase-5 inhibitor used to treat erectile dysfunction and pulmonary arterial hypertension [82]. Several studies have demonstrated that this drug reduces the activation of platelet-dependent glycoprotein IIb/IIIa in patients with SCD and pulmonary hypertension [83]. Sildenafil also increases the signalization of cGMP signaling which could be useful in the treatment of SCD patients with pulmonary hypertension [84, 85].

Statins efficiently prevent blood vessel damage *via* many mechanisms, including by increasing endothelial NO. These drugs also reduce vascular inflammation and restore endothelial relaxation in coronary diseases and stroke. Some studies have reported that lovastatin reduces the expression of platelet activation factor on the vascular endothelium [86].

Adenosine agonists

Adenosine is an endogenous purine nucleoside, whose signaling is responsible for promoting vasodilation, reducing inflammation, and protecting tissues during periods of hypoxia and

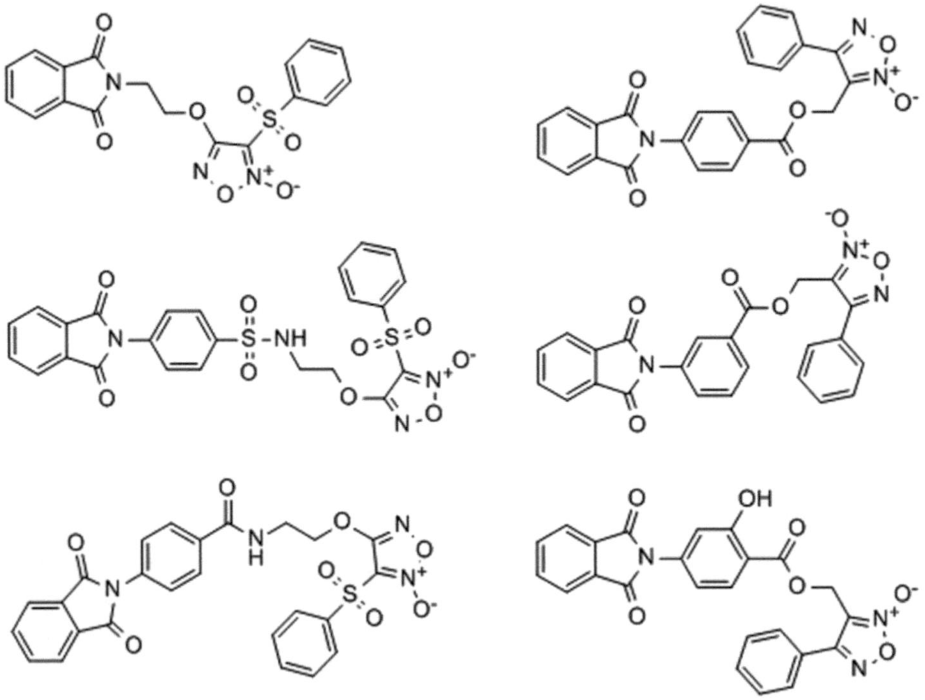

Figure 11. Furoxan derivatives with NO-donor ability.

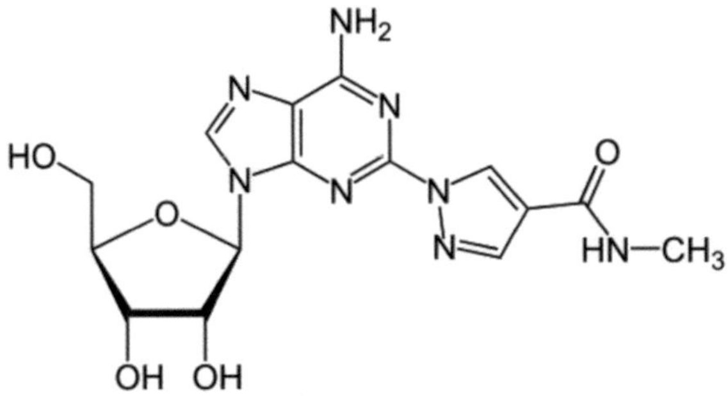

Figure 12. Chemical structure of regadenoson.

cellular stress [87]. In SCD patients, the tissue damage generated by ischemia–reperfusion may reduce the plasma levels of adenosine [88].

Some studies have suggested that receptors A_{2A} and A_{2B} are related to the pathogenesis of SCD. ATL146e is an A_{2A} adenosine agonist that reduces the activation of leukocytes, platelets, and invariant natural killer T cells (iNKT cells), inflammation, and pulmonary injury in transgenic animals with SCD [89]. Regadenoson (Figure 12) is a selective agonist of the A_{2a} adenosine receptor. During clinical trials (phase I), this compound reduced the activation of iNKT cells, with no toxic effects [90].

It has been reported that the activation of the adenosine A_{2B} receptor may increase the deleterious effects of SCD, promoting priapism and the sickling of erythrocytes [91]. Antagonists such as MS-1706 can reverse priapism [92]. Therefore, the adenosine signaling pathway is a promising target for the treatment of SCD. A double therapy with an A2A agonist and an A2B antagonist could have beneficial effects in patients, reducing inflammation, sickling, and priapism. However, more studies are required to understand the beneficial effects of these compounds in the treatment of SCD.

Hemoglobin modifiers

The hemoglobin modifiers are classified as either covalent or noncovalent. Although noncovalent modifiers have shown interesting activities, their use is still limited [93]. The modification of hemoglobin by covalent modifiers reduces erythrocyte sickling by two possible mechanisms: by increasing HbS solubility and/or by increasing its affinity for oxygen [94].

Isothiocyanates have been described as potential modifiers of HbS solubility, delaying its polymerization, specifically because they bind to the β subunit of HbS, which is responsible for the hydrophobic interactions that result in its polymerization [95].

Aldehyde compounds have the capacity to form adducts (Schiff bases) with the N-terminal amines on the amino acids in the HbS chain. Safo et al (2004) demonstrated that heterocyclic aldehydes, such as furfural, 5-methylfurfural, 5-ethylfurfural, and 5-hydroxymethylfurfural, increase the affinity of HbS for oxygen, thereby inhibiting sickling [96]. However, the low oral bioavailability of these drugs, the high doses required for a significant effect, and their dose-dependent toxicity limit their therapeutic use.

Rho-kinase (ROCK) inhibitors

The Rho-kinase protein (ROCK), identified as a Rho-GTPase effector, is involved in various cell processes, including contractility, chemotaxis, adhesion, and migration. This protein facilitates the infiltration of inflammatory cells, both *in vitro* and *in vivo* [97].

ROCK inhibition is beneficial in cardiovascular, neurological, and oncological diseases. The *in vivo* activities of these inhibitors include: a) the regulation of the arterial blood pressure; b) increased vascular resistance; c) the regression of atherosclerotic coronary lesions; d) the prevention of diabetes development; e) neurological repair; f) reduced formation of β-myeloid aggregates; and g) the inhibition of tumor growth, progression, and metastasis [98-105].

Rho-kinase inhibitors are also potential agents for the treatment of SCD. An *in vitro* study showed that Rho-kinase inhibitors, such as Y-27632 (Figure 13), reduced the activation of human endothelial cells and the adhesion of eosinophils in SCD patients. Fasudil (Figure 13) is a Rho-kinase inhibitor that is approved in Japan for the treatment and prevention of intracranial aneurysm and that has shown good results in preventing pulmonary complications in animals with SCD. The activities of fasudil include: a) the inhibition of eosinophil and chemokine recruitment, which promotes the progression of the pulmonary inflammatory response [106]; b) the reduction of proinflammatory cytokines levels, such as IL-6, IL1-β, and TNF-α, thus reducing inflammation [107]; and c) the reduction of the expression of adhesive molecules, such as ICAM-1, and therefore coagulation [108].

A comparison of HU and hydroxyfasudil demonstrated the superior activity of the ROCK inhibitor in reducing vaso-occlusion and inflammation. Therefore, this class of drug has been suggested as an alternative SCD treatment [109].

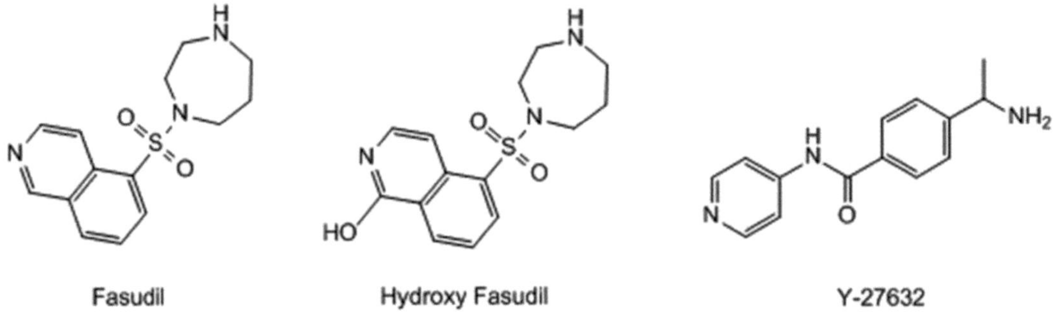

Figure 13. Chemical structures of Rho-kinase inhibitors.

Chelating agents

Iron-chelation therapies have been used to control iron overload in patients who have received several blood transfusions to reduce disease complications [110]. Iron overload can affect organs such as the liver, heart, and endocrine system, leading to tissue damage and even death [111].

Deferoxamine is a hexadentate chelating agent, introduced into the therapeutic context in 1963. It is still one of the drugs most frequently used to treat iron overload in hemoglobin disorders, such as SCD and thalassemia. Deferoxamine has a high molecular weight and a high affinity for Fe^{3+}, and the ratio between the drug and iron is 1:1. Because this drug has low oral/gastrointestinal absorption, it is administered *via* a subcutaneous or intravenous route [112].

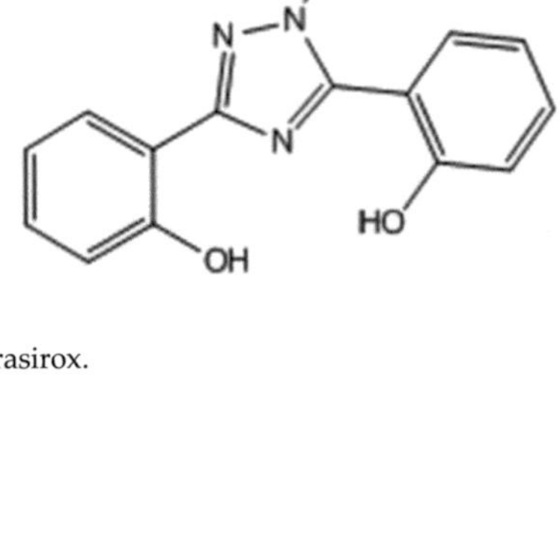

Figure 14. Chemical structure of deferasirox.

Deferasirox was approved by the FDA in November 2005 as an oral chelating agent. It is a trivalent molecule with great affinity for the iron atom. The chelating ratio is two drug molecules to each iron atom (Figure 14) [113]. The prolonged chelating effect produces a progressive reduction in free plasma iron. Its oral route of administration is the great advantage of this drug, but the treatment is expensive [114].

2. Conclusions

Sickle cell disease is one of the most prevalent hemoglobinopathies worldwide. Despite its importance, therapeutic resources are scarce and usually only control the main symptoms of the disease. The lack of interest by pharmaceutical companies in developing new drugs for SCD and the limited research undertaken in this area ensure that this disease still severely affects patients. The only drug currently available to treat SCD is HU, but its serious adverse effects limit its use. Moreover, around 1/3 of patients do not respond to HU treatment.

Therefore, research is urgently required to find new drugs for SCD. In this chapter, we have discussed the currently available treatments and their limitations, and have presented and discussed new approaches. Among these, the adenosine agonists/antagonists and ROCK inhibitors seem the most promising strategies, and therefore warrant further investigation.

Acknowledgements

This study was supported by Fundacão de Amparo à Pesquisa do Estado de São Paulo (FAPESP ref. Process: 2012/50359-2 and 2014/06755-6), PADC-FCF -UNESP.

Author details

Thais Regina Ferreira de Melo[1], Lucas dos Reis Ercolin[1], Rafael Consolin Chelucci[1], Aylime Castanho Bolognesi Melchior[1], Carolina Lanaro[2], Chung Man Chin[1] and Jean Leandro dos Santos[1*]

*Address all correspondence to: santosjl@fcfar.unesp.br

1 School of Pharmaceutical Science - State University of São Paulo (UNESP), Araraquara, São Paulo, Brazil

2 The Haematology and Haemotherapy Centre, University of Campinas—UNICAMP, Campinas, São Paulo, Brazil

References

[1] Weatherall DJ. Genetic variation and susceptibility to infection: The red cell and malaria. British Journal of Haematology. 2008;141(3):276–286.

[2] Taylor SM, Parobek CM, Fairhurst RM. Haemoglobinopathies and the clinical epidemiology of malaria: A systematic review and meta-analysis. The Lancet Infectious Diseases. 2012;12(6):457–468.

[3] Min-Oo G, Gros P. Erythrocyte variants and the nature of their malaria protective effect. Cellular Microbiology. 2005; 7(6):753–763.

[4] Piel FB, Patil AP, Howes RE, Nyangiri O A, Gething PW, Williams TN, Weatherall DJ, Hay SI. Global distribution of the sickle cell gene and geographical confirmation of the malaria hypothesis. Nature communications. 2010;1:104.

[5] Gong L, Parikh S, Rosenthal PJ, Greenhouse B. Biochemical and immunological mechanisms by which sickle cell trait protects against malaria. Malaria journal. 2013;12(1): 317.

[6] Bonds DR. Three decades of innovation in the management of sickle cell disease: The road to understanding the sickle cell disease clinical phenotype. Blood Reviews. 2005; 19(2):99–110.

[7] Simões BP, Pieroni F, Barros GMN, Machado CL, Cançado RD, Salvino MA, Angulo I, Voltarelli JC. Brazilian Consensus Meeting on Stem Cell Transplantation: Hemoglobinopathies Committee. Revista Brasileira de Hematologia e Hemoterapia. 2010; 32(1):46–53.

[8] Vespoli S, Marques M, Marane SSG, Santos VF, Chung MC, Santos JL. Análise das prevalências de doenças detectadas pelo programa nacional de triagem neonatal no município de Araraquara no ano de 2009. Revista de Ciências Farmacêuticas Básica e Aplicada. 2011;32(2):269–273.

[9] Bunn HF. Pathogenesis and Treatment of Sickle Cell Disease. The New England Journal of Medicine. 1997;337(11):762–769.

[10] De Franceschi L, Corrocher R. Established and experimental treatments for sickle cell disease. Haematologica. 2004;89(3):348–356.

[11] Rees DC, Williams TN, Gladwin MT. Sickle-cell disease. The Lancet. 2010; 376(9757): 2018–2031.

[12] Brittenham GM, Griffith PM, Nienhuis AW, McLaren CE, Young NS, Tucker EE, Allen CJ, Farrell DE, Harris JW. Efficacy of deferoxamine in preventing complications of iron overload in patients with thalassemia major. The New England journal of medicine. 1994;331(9):567–573.

[13] Reiter CD, Wang X, Tanus-Santos JE, Hogg N, Cannon RO, Schechter AN, Gladwin MT. Cell-free hemoglobin limits nitric oxide bioavailability in sickle-cell disease. Nature medicine. 2002;8(12):1383–1389.

[14] Rother RP, Bell L, Hillmen P. The clinical sequelae of intravascular hemolysis and extracellular plasma hemoglobin: A novel mechanism of human disease. The Journal of the American Medical Association. 2005;293(13):1653–1662.

[15] Kato GJ, McGowan V, Machado RF, Little JA, Taylor VI J, Morris CR, Nichols JS, Wang X, Poljakovic M, Morris SM, Gladwin MT. Lactate dehydrogenase as a biomarker of hemolysis-associated nitric oxide resistance, priapism, leg ulceration, pulmonary hypertension, and death in patients with sickle cell disease. Blood. 2006;107(6):2279–2285.

[16] Conran N, Oresco-Santos C, Acosta HC, Fattori A, Saad STO, Costa FF. Increased soluble guanylate cyclase activity in the red blood cells of sickle cell patients. British Journal of Haematology. 2004;124(4):547–554.

[17] Cokic VP, Smith RD, Beleslin-cokic BB, Njoroge JM, Miller JL, Gladwin MT, Schechter AN. Hydroxyurea induces fetal hemoglobin by the nitric oxide – dependent activation of soluble guanylyl cyclase. Journal of Clinical Investigation. 2003;111(2):231–239.

[18] Sakamoto TM, Lanaro C, Ozelo MC, Garrido VT, Olalla-Saad ST, Conran N, Costa FF. Increased adhesive and inflammatory properties in blood outgrowth endothelial cells from sickle cell anemia patients. Microvascular Research. 2013;90:173–179.

[19] Zennadi R, Chien A, Xu K, Batchvarova M, Telen MJ. Sickle red cells induce adhesion of lymphocytes and monocytes to endothelium. Blood. 2008;112(8):3474–3483.

[20] Kaul DK, Finnegan E, Barabino G a. Sickle red cell-endothelium interactions. Microcirculation. 2009;16(1):97–111.

[21] Belcher JD, Mahaseth H, Welch TE, Vilback AE, Sonbol KM, Kalambur VS, Bowlin PR, Bischof JC, Hebbel RP, Vercellotti GM. Critical role of endothelial cell activation in hypoxia-induced vasoocclusion in transgenic sickle mice. American journal of physiology Heart and circulatory physiology. 2005;288(6):2715–2725.

[22] Wood KC, Hebbel RP, Granger DN. Endothelial cell NADPH oxidase mediates the cerebral microvascular dysfunction in sickle cell transgenic mice. The FASEB journal. 2005;19(8):989–991.

[23] Perelman N, Selvaraj SK, Batra S, Luck LR, Erdreich-epstein A, Coates TD, Kalra VK, Malik P. Placenta growth factor activates monocytes and correlates with sickle cell disease severity. Growth. 2003;102(4):1506–1514.

[24] Okpala I. The intriguing contribution of white blood cells to sickle cell disease - A red cell disorder. Blood Reviews. 2004;18(1):65–73.

[25] Malavé I, Perdomo Y, Escalona E, Rodriguez E, Anchustegui M, Malavé H AT. Levels of tumor necrosis factor alpha/cachectin (TNF alpha) in sera from patients with sickle cell disease. Acta Haematologica. 1993;90(4):172–176.

[26] Lanaro C, Franco-Penteado CF, Albuqueque DM, Saad STO, Conran N, Costa FF. Altered levels of cytokines and inflammatory mediators in plasma and leukocytes of sickle cell anemia patients and effects of hydroxyurea therapy. Journal of leukocyte biology. 2009;85(2):235–242.

[27] Inglis JJ, Nissim A, Lees DM, Hunt SP, Chernajovsky Y, Kidd BL. The differential contribution of tumour necrosis factor to thermal and mechanical hyperalgesia during chronic inflammation. Arthritis research & therapy. 2005;7(4):807–816.

[28] Francis RB, Haywood LJ. Elevated immunoreactive tumor necrosis factor and interleukin-1 in sickle cell disease. Journal of the National Medical Association. 1992;84(7): 611–615.

[29] Buchanan GR, DeBaun MR, Quinn CT, Steinberg MH. Sickle cell disease. Hematology. 2004;2004(1):35–47.

[30] O'Connell D. Neglected Diseases. Nature. 2007;449:157.

[31] Gee BE. Biologic complexity in sickle cell disease: Implications for developing targeted therapeutics. ScientificWorldJournal. 2013; 694146.

[32] Steinberg, MH, Rodgers GP. Pharmacologic Modulation of Fetal Hemoglobin. Medicine. 2001;80(5):328–344.

[33] Pace BS, Zein S. Understanding mechanisms of gamma-globin gene regulation to develop strategies for pharmacological fetal hemoglobin induction. Developmental Dynamics. 2006;235(7):1727–1737.

[34] Platt OS; Brambilla DJ; Rosse WF; Milner PF; Castro O; Steinberg MH; Klug PP. Mortality in sickle cell disease. Life expectancy and risk factors for early death. New England Journal of Medicine. 1994;330(23):1639–1644.

[35] Akinsheye I, Alsultan A, Solovieff N, Ngo D, Baldwin CT, Sebastiani P, Chui DHK, Steinberg MH. Fetal hemoglobin in sickle cell anemia. Blood. 2011;118(1):19–27.

[36] Hanft VN, Fruchtman SR, Pickens C V, Rosse WF, Howard TA, Ware RE. Acquired DNA mutations associated with in vivo hydroxyurea exposure. Blood. 2000;95(11): 3589–3593.

[37] Charache S, Terrin ML, Moore RD, Dover GJ, Barton FB, Eckert SV, McMahon RP, Bonds DR. Effect of hydroxyurea on the frequency of painful crises in sickle cell anemia. Investigators of the Multicenter Study of Hydroxyurea in Sickle Cell Anemia. The New England Journal of Medicine. 1995;332(20):1317–1322.

[38] Ferster a, Tahriri P, Vermylen C, Sturbois G, Corazza F, Fondu P, Devalck C, Dresse MF, Feremans W, Hunninck K, Toppet M, Philippet P, Van Geet C, Sariban E. Five

years of experience with hydroxyurea in children and young adults with sickle cell disease. Blood. 2001;97(11):3628–3632.

[39] Cokic VP, Andric SA, Stojilkovic SS, Noguchi CT, Schechter AN. Hydroxyurea nitrosylates and activates soluble guanylyl cyclase in human erythroid cells. Blood. 2008; 111(3):1117–1123.

[40] Hillery CA, Du MC, Wang WC, Scott JP. Hydroxyurea therapy decreases the in vitro adhesion of sickle erythrocytes to thrombospondin and laminin. British Journal of Haematology. 2000;109(2):322–327.

[41] Nahavandi M, Tavakkoli F, Wyche MQ, Perlin E, Winter WP, Castro O. Nitric oxide and cyclic GMP levels in sickle cell patients receiving hydroxyurea. British Journal of Haematology. 2002;119(3):855–857.

[42] Raghupathy R, Billett HH. Promising therapies in sickle cell disease. Cardiovascular & hematological disorders drug targets. 2009;9(1):1–8.

[43] Moncada S HA. The L-Arginine-Nitric Oxide Pathway. New England Journal of Medicine. 1993;329(27):2002–2012.

[44] Nathan C, Xie Q. Nitric oxide synthases: rolls, tolls and controls. Cell. 1994;78(6):915–918.

[45] Reiter CD, Gladwin MT. An emerging role for nitric oxide in sickle cell disease vascular homeostasis and therapy. Current opinion in hematology. 2003;10(2):99–107.

[46] Stamler JS, Simon DI, Osborne JA, Mullins ME, Jaraki O, Michel T, Singel DJ, Loscalzo J. S-nitrosylation of proteins with nitric oxide: synthesis and characterization of biologically active compounds. Proceedings of the National Academy of Sciences of the United States of America. 1992;89(1):444–448.

[47] Illi B, Colussi C, Grasselli A, Farsetti A, Capogrossi MC, Gaetano C. NO sparks off chromatin: Tales of a multifaceted epigenetic regulator. Pharmacology and Therapeutics. 2009;123(3):344–352.

[48] Nott A, Watson PM, Robinson JD, Crepaldi L, Riccio A. S-Nitrosylation of histone deacetylase 2 induces chromatin remodelling in neurons. Nature. 2008;455(7211): 411–415.

[49] DeSimone J, Heller P, Schimenti JC, Duncan CH. Fetal hemoglobin production in adult baboons by 5-azacytidine or by phenylhydrazine-induced hemolysis is associated with hypomethylation of globin gene DNA. Progress in clinical and biological research. 1983;134 489–500.

[50] Saunthararajah Y, Hillery CA, Lavelle D, Molokie R, Dorn L, Bressler L, Gavazova S, Chen Y, Hoffman R, Desimone J. Effects of 5-aza-2'-deoxycytidine on fetal hemoglobin levels, red cell adhesion, and hematopoietic differentiation in patients with sickle cell disease. Hemoglobin. 2003;102(12):3865–3870.

[51] Lantry LE, Zhang Z, Crist K a, Wang Y, Kelloff GJ, Lubet R a, You M. 5-Aza-2′-deoxycytidine is chemopreventive in a 4-(methyl-nitrosamino)-1-(3-pyridyl)-1-butanone-induced primary mouse lung tumor model. Carcinogenesis. 1999;20(2):343–346.

[52] Santos JL, Chin CM. Recent insights on the medicinal chemistry of sickle cell disease. Current Medicinal Chemistry. 2011;18(15):2339–2358.

[53] Carr BI, Reilly JG, Smith SS, Winberg C, Riggs A. The tumorigenicity of 5-azacytidine in the male Fischer rat. Carcinogenesis. 1984;5(12):1583–1590.

[54] McCaffrey PG, Newsome DA, Fibach E, Yoshida M, Su MSS. Induction of gamma-globin by histone deacetylase inhibitors. Blood. 1997;90(5):2075–2083.

[55] Kutlar A, Ataga K, Reid M, Vichinsky EP, Neumayr L, Blair-Britt L, Labotka R, Glass J, Keefer JR, Wargin WA, Berenson R, Perrine SP. A Phase 1/2 Trial of HQK-1001, an Oral Fetal Globin Inducer, in Sickle Cell Disease. American Journal of Hematology. 2012;87(11):1017–1021.

[56] Little JA,, Vicki R. McGowan, Gregory J. Kato, Kristine S. Partovi JJF, Irina Maric, Sabrina Martyr, James G. Taylor VI, Roberto F. Machado TH, Oswaldo Castro, Gladwin MT. Combination Erythropoietin-Hydroxyurea Therapy in Sickle Cell Disease: NIH experience and literature review. Haematologica. 2006;91(8):1076–1083.

[57] Mcbride WG. Thalidomide and Congenital Abnormalities. The Lancet. 1961;278(7216):1358.

[58] Eriksson T, Björkman S, Höglund P. Clinical pharmacology of thalidomide. European Journal of Clinical Pharmacology. 2001;57(5):365–376.

[59] Aerbajinai W, Zhu J, Gao Z, Chin K, Rodgers GP. Thalidomide induces gamma-globin gene expression through increased reactive oxygen species mediated p38 MAPK signaling and histone H4 acetylation in adult erythropoiesis. Blood. 2007;110(8):2864–2871.

[60] Hsiao CH, Li W, Lou TF, Baliga BS, Pace BS. Fetal hemoglobin induction by histone deacetylase inhibitors involves generation of reactive oxygen species. Experimental hematology. 2006;34(3):264–273.

[61] List A, Dewald G, Bennett J, Giagounidis A, Raza A, Feldman E, Powell B, Greenberg P, Thomas D, Stone R, Reeder C, Wride K, Patin J, Schmidt M, Zeldis J, Knight R. Lenalidomide in the myelodysplastic syndrome with chromosome 5q deletion. The New England journal of medicine. 2006;355(14):1456–1465.

[62] Moutouh-De Parseval LA, Verhelle D, Glezer E, Jensen-Pergakes K, Ferguson GD, Corral LG, Morris CL, Muller G, Brady H, Chan K. Pomalidomide and lenalidomide regulate erythropoiesis and fetal hemoglobin production in human CD34+ cells. Journal of Clinical Investigation. 2008;118(1):248–258.

[63] Meiler SE, Wade M, Kutlar F, Yerigenahally SD, Xue Y, Moutouh-De Parseval LA, Corral LG, Swerdlow PS, Kutlar A. Pomalidomide augments fetal hemoglobin pro-

duction without the myelosuppressive effects of hydroxyurea in transgenic sickle cell mice. Blood. 2011;118(4):1109–1112.

[64] Flatman PW. Regulation of Na-K-2Cl cotransport in red cells. Advances in experimental medicine and biology. 2004;559:77–88.

[65] Lew VL, Tiffert T, Etzion Z, Perdomo D, Daw N, Macdonald L, Bookchin RM. Distribution of dehydration rates generated by maximal Gardos-channel activation in normal and sickle red blood cells. Blood. 2005;105(1):361–367.

[66] Brugnara C TD. Inhibition of K transport by divalent cations in sickle erythrocytes. Blood. 1987;70(6):1810–1815.

[67] De Franceschi L, Saadane N, Trudel M, Alper SL, Brugnara C, Beuzard Y. Treatment with oral clotrimazole blocks Ca(2+)-activated K+ transport and reverses erythrocyte dehydration in transgenic SAD mice: A model for therapy of sickle cell disease. Journal of Clinical Investigation. 1994;93(10):1670–1676.

[68] Hankins J, Aygun B. Pharmacotherapy in sickle cell disease - State of the art and future prospects. British Journal of Haematology. 2009;145(3):296–308.

[69] Bennekou P, De Franceschi L, Pedersen O, Lian L, Asakura T, Evans G, Brugnara C, Christophersen P. Treatment with NS3623, a novel Cl-conductance blocker, ameliorates erythrocyte dehydration in transgenic SAD mice: A possible new therapeutic approach for sickle cell disease. Blood. 2001;97(5):1451–1457.

[70] McNaughton-Smith G a., Burns JF, Stocker JW, Rigdon GC, Creech C, Arlington S, Shelton T, De Franceschi L. Novel inhibitors of the gardos channel for the treatment of sickle cell disease. Journal of Medicinal Chemistry. 2008;51(4):976–982.

[71] Stocker JW, De Franceschi L, McNaughton-Smith G a., Corrocher R, Beuzard Y, Brugnara C. ICA-17043, a novel Gardos channel blocker, prevents sickled red blood cell dehydration in vitro and in vivo in SAD mice. Blood. 2003;101(6):2412–2418.

[72] Embury SH, Matsui NM, Ramanujam S, Mayadas TN, Noguchi CT, Diwan B a., Mohandas N, Cheung ATW. The contribution of endothelial cell P-selectin to the microvascular flow of mouse sickle erythrocytes in vivo. Blood. 2004;104(10):3378–3385.

[73] Matsui NM, Varki A, Embury SH. Heparin inhibits the flow adhesion of sickle red blood cells to P-selectin. Blood. 2002;100(10):3790–3796.

[74] Chang J, Patton JT, Sarkar A, Ernst B, Magnani JL, Frenette PS. GMI-1070, a novel pan-selectin antagonist, reverses acute vascular occlusions in sickle cell mice. Blood. 2010; 116(10):1779–1786.

[75] Lee SP, Ataga KI, Zayed M, Manganello JM, Orringer EP, Phillips DR, Parise L V. Phase I study of eptifibatide in patients with sickle cell anaemia. British Journal of Haematology. 2007;139(4):612–620.

[76] Mack a K, Kato GJ. Sickle cell disease and nitric oxide: a paradigm shift? International Journal of Biochemistry & Cell Biology. 2006;38(8):1237–1243.

[77] Atz AM WD. Inhaled nitric oxide in sickle cell disease with acute chest syndrome. Anesthesiology. 1997;87(4):988–990.

[78] Santos JL, Lanaro C, Chelucci RC, Gambero S, Bosquesi PL, Reis JS, Lima LM, Cerecetto H, González M, Costa FF, Chung MC. Design, synthesis, and pharmacological evaluation of novel hybrid compounds to treat sickle cell disease symptoms. Part II: Furoxan derivatives. Journal of Medicinal Chemistry. 2012;55(17):7583–7592.

[79] Santos JL, Lanaro C, Lima LM, Gambero S, Franco-Penteado CF, Alexandre-Moreira MS, Wade M, Yerigenahally S, Kutlar A, Meiler SE, Costa FF, Chung M. Design, synthesis, and pharmacological evaluation of novel hybrid compounds to treat sickle cell disease symptoms. Journal of Medicinal Chemistry. 2011;54(16):5811–5819.

[80] Morris CR, Kuypers FA, Larkin S, Vichinsky EP, Styles LA. Patterns of arginine and nitric oxide in patients with sickle cell disease with vaso-occlusive crisis and acute chest syndrome. Journal of pediatric hematology/oncology. 2000;22(6):515–520.

[81] Morris CR, Morris SM, Hagar W, Van Warmerdam J, Claster S, Kepka-Lenhart D, Machado L, Kuypers F a., Vichinsky EP. Arginine therapy: A new treatment for pulmonary hypertension in sickle cell disease? American Journal of Respiratory and Critical Care Medicine. 2003;168(1):63–69.

[82] Atz AM, Wessel DL. Sildenafil ameliorates effects of inhaled nitric oxide withdrawal. Anesthesiology. 1999;91(1):307–310.

[83] Villagra J, Shiva S, Hunter L a., Machado RF, Gladwin MT, Kato GJ. Platelet activation in patients with sickle disease, hemolysis-associated pulmonary hypertension, and nitric oxide scavenging by cell-free hemoglobin. Blood. 2007;110(6):2166–2172.

[84] Burnett AL, Bivalacqua TJ, Champion HC, Musicki B. Long-term oral phosphodiesterase 5 inhibitor therapy alleviates recurrent priapism. Urology. 2006;67(5):1043–1048.

[85] Bialecki E, Bridges K. Sildenafil relives priapism in patients with sickle cell disease. The American Journal of Medicine. 2002;113(3):252.

[86] Solovey A, Kollander R, Shet A, Milbauer LC, Choong S, Panoskaltsis-Mortari A, Blazar BR, Kelm Jr RJ, Hebbel RP. Endothelial cell expression of tissue factor in sickle mice is augmented by hypoxia / reoxygenation and inhibited by lovastatin Endothelial cell expression of tissue factor in sickle mice is augmented by hypoxia / reoxygenation and inhibited by lovastatin. Cell. 2008;104(3):840–846.

[87] Jacobson KA, Gao ZG. Adenosine receptors as therapeutic targets. Nature Review Drug Discovery. 2006;5(3):247–264.

[88] Field JJ, Nathan DG, Linden J. The role of adenosine signaling in sickle cell therapeutics. Hematology/Oncology Clinics of North America. 2014;28(2):287–299.

[89] Wallace KL, Linden J. Adenosine A 2A receptors induced on iNKT and NK cells reduce pulmonary inflammation and injury in mice with sickle cell disease. Electronics. 2010;116(23):5010–5020.

[90] Field JJ, Lin G, Okam MM, Majerus E, Keefer J, Onyekwere O, Ross A, Campigotto F, Neuberg D, Linden J, Nathan DG. Sickle cell vaso-occlusion causes activation of iNKT cells that is decreased by the adenosine A 2A receptor agonist regadenoson Sickle cell vaso-occlusion causes activation of iNKT cells that is decreased by the adenosine A 2A receptor agonist regadenoson. Blood. 2013;121(17):3329–3334.

[91] Zhang Y, Dai Y, Wen J, Zhang W, Grenz A, Sun H, Tao L, Lu G, Alexander DC, Milburn M V, Carter-Dawson L, Lewis DE, Zhang W, Eltzschig HK, Kellems RE, Blackburn MR, Juneja HS, Xia Y. Detrimental effects of adenosine signaling in sickle cell disease. Nature medicine. 2011;17(1):79–86.

[92] Mi T, Abbasi S, Zhang H, Uray K, Chunn JL, Ling WX, Molina JG, Weisbrodt NW, Kellems RE, Blackburn MR, Xia Y. Excess adenosine in murine penile erectile tissues contributes to priapism via A2B adenosine receptor signaling. Journal of Clinical Investigation. 2008;118(4):1491–1501.

[93] Waterman MR, Yamaoka K, Dahm L, Taylor J, Cottam GL. Noncovalent modification of deoxyhemoglobin S solubility and erythrocyte sickling. Proceedings of the National Academy of Sciences of the United States of America. 1974;71(6):2222–2225.

[94] Ueno H, Bai Y, Manning JM. Covalent chemical modifiers of sickle cell hemoglobin. Annals of the New York Academy of Sciences. 1989;565:239–246.

[95] Park S, Hayes BL, Marankan F, Mulhearn DC, Wanna L, Mesecar AD, Santarsiero BD, Johnson ME, Venton DL. Regioselective covalent modification of hemoglobin in search of antisickling agents. Journal of Medicinal Chemistry. 2003;46(6):936–953.

[96] Safo MK, Abdulmalik O, Danso-Danquah R, Burnett JC, Nokuri S, Joshi GS, Musayev FN, Asakura T, Abraham DJ. Structural basis for the potent antisickling effect of a novel class of five-membered heterocyclic aldehydic compounds. Journal of Medicinal Chemistry. 2004;47(19):4665–4676.

[97] Boureux A, Vignal E, Faure S, Fort P. Evolution of the Rho family of Ras-like GTPases in eukaryotes. Molecular Biology and Evolution. 2007;24(1):203–216.

[98] Fukumoto Y, Matoba T, Ito A, Tanaka H, Kishi T, Hayashidani S, Abe K, Takeshita A, Shimokawa H. Acute vasodilator effects of a Rho-kinase inhibitor, fasudil, in patients with severe pulmonary hypertension. Heart. 2005;91(3):391–392.

[99] Kandabashi T, Shimokawa H, Miyata K, Kunihiro I, Kawano Y, Fukata Y, Higo T, Egashira K, Takahashi S, Kaibuchi K, Takeshita A. Inhibition of myosin phosphatase

by upregulated rho-kinase plays a key role for coronary artery spasm in a porcine model with interleukin-1beta. Circulation. 2000;101(11):1319–1323.

[100] Shimokawa H, Morishige K, Miyata K, Kandabashi T, Eto Y, Ikegaki I, Asano T, Kaibuchi K, Takeshita A. Long-term inhibition of Rho-kinase induces a regression of arteriosclerotic coronary lesions in a porcine model in vivo. Cardiovascular Research. 2001;51(1):169–177.

[101] Kishi T, Hirooka Y, Masumoto A, Ito K, Kimura Y, Inokuchi K, Tagawa T, Shimokawa H, Takeshita A, Sunagawa K. Rho-kinase inhibitor improves increased vascular resistance and impaired vasodilation of the forearm in patients with heart failure. Circulation. 2005;111(21):2741–2747.

[102] Hara M, Takayasu M, Watanabe K, Noda A, Takagi T, Suzuki Y, Yoshida J. Protein kinase inhibition by fasudil hydrochloride promotes neurological recovery after spinal cord injury in rats. Journal of Neurosurgery. 2000;93(1):94–101.

[103] Song Y, Chen X, Wang LY, Gao W, Zhu MJ. Rho kinase inhibitor fasudil protects againstbeta-amyloid-induced hippocampal neurodegeneration in rats. CNS Neuroscience and Therapeutics. 2013;19(8):603–610.

[104] Liu J, Obando D, Schipanski LG, Groebler LK, Witting PK, Kalinowski DS, Richardson DR, Codd R. Conjugates of desferrioxamine B (DFOB) with derivatives of adamantane or with orally available chelators as potential agents for treating iron overload. Journal of Medicinal Chemistry. 2010;53(3):1370–1382.

[105] Ying H, Biroc SL, Li W-W, Alicke B, Xuan J-A, Pagila R, Ohashi Y, Okada T, Kamata Y, Dinter H. The Rho kinase inhibitor fasudil inhibits tumor progression in human and rat tumor models. Molecular cancer therapeutics. 2006;5(9):2158–2164.

[106] Pallis FR, Vital MD, Fertrin KY, Saad STO, Conran N, Costa FF, Franco-Penteado CF. Inhibition Of the Rho/Rho-Kinase Pathway Reduces In Vitro Adhesion Of Sickle Cell Anemia Eosinophils To Human Endothelial Cells. Blood. 2013;122(21):2219.

[107] Ding J, Li QY, Wang X, Sun CH, Lu CZ, Xiao BG. Fasudil protects hippocampal neurons against hypoxia-reoxygenation injury by suppressing microglial inflammatory responses in mice. Journal of Neurochemistry. 2010;114(6):1619–1629.

[108] Washida N, Wakino S, Tonozuka Y, Homma K, Tokuyama H, Hara Y, Hasegawa K, Minakuchi H, Fujimura K, Hosoya K, Hayashi K, Itoh H. Rho-kinase inhibition ameliorates peritoneal fibrosis and angiogenesis in a rat model of peritoneal sclerosis. Nephrology Dialysis Transplantation. 2011;26(9):2770–2779.

[109] Essack M, Radovanovic A, Bajic VB. Information Exploration System for Sickle Cell Disease and Repurposing of Hydroxyfasudil. PLoS ONE. 2013; 8(6):e65190.

[110] Wanko SO, Telen MJ. Transfusion management in sickle cell disease. Hematology/Oncology Clinics of North America. 2005;19(5):803–826.

[111] Raghupathy R, Manwani D, Little J a. Iron overload in sickle cell disease. Advances in hematology. 2010;2010:272940.

[112] Kontoghiorghes GJ, Eracleous E, Economides C, Kolnagou A. Advances in iron overload therapies. Prospects for effective use of deferiprone (L1), deferoxamine, the new experimental chelators ICL670, GT56-252, L1NA11 and their combinations. Current Medicinal Chemistry. 2005;12(23):2663–2681.

[113] Porter JB. Deferasirox - Current knowledge and future challenges. Annals of the New York Academy of Sciences. 2010;1202:87–93.

[114] Séchaud R, Robeva A, Belleli R, Balez S. Absolute oral bioavailability and disposition of deferasirox in healthy human subjects. Journal of Clinical Pharmacology. 2008;48(8):919–925.